I0466766

CRPS

DIET COOKBOOK FOR BEGINNERS

Delicious and Nutritious Recipes for Pain Relief, Healing, and Improved Well-Being

Kingsley Klopp

To show our appreciation for your purchase, we're delighted to offer you these special bonuses as a heartfelt thank you.

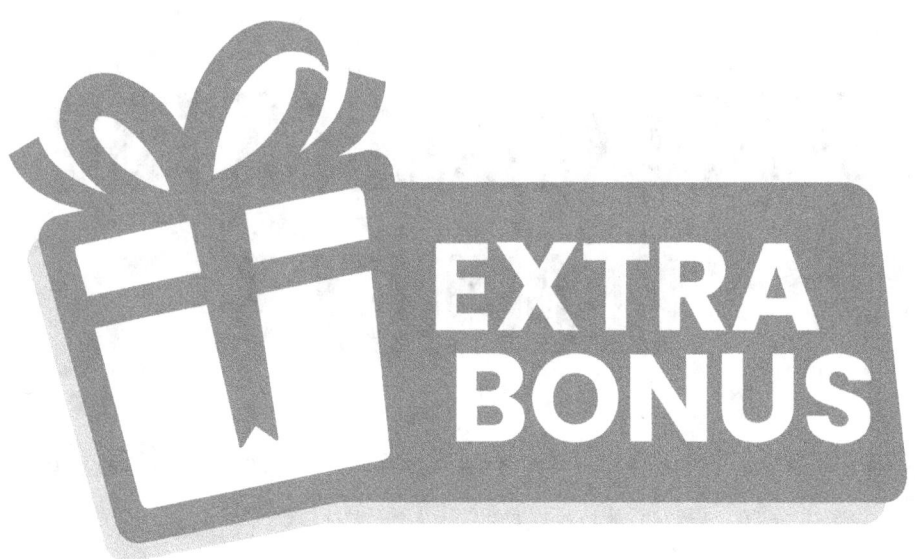

1. A Food Tracker Journal
2. Downloadable E-BOOK featuring full-color images of finished recipes

Copyright © 2024 All rights reserved.

No part of this book may be reproduced or transmitted in any form or by any means, electronic or mechanical, including photocopying, recording, or by any information storage and retrieval system, without written permission from the author. The scanning, uploading, and distribution of this book via the internet or via any other means without the permission of the author is illegal and punishable by law. The author has made every effort to ensure the accuracy of the information contained in this book. However, the author cannot be held responsible for any errors or omissions.

Table of Contents

Poultry Recipes

Meat Recipes

Fish & Seafood Recipes

Soup & Stew Recipes

Important Note

Thank you for choosing the **Complex Regional Pain Syndrome (CRPS) Diet Cookbook.** We are thrilled to have you join us on this culinary journey towards better health and well-being. Before you dive into the delicious recipes and nutritious meals we've crafted, we want to share an important note. Everyone's body is unique, and what works wonders for one person might not have the same effect for another. CRPS can manifest differently in each individual, and your dietary needs may vary based on a variety of factors, including other health conditions, allergies, and personal preferences. Therefore, we encourage you to treat this cookbook as a flexible guide rather than a rigid rulebook. Feel free to adjust the recipes to suit your personal needs and taste.

It's also crucial to consult with your healthcare provider before making significant changes to your diet, especially if you have any concerns or questions. Your doctor can provide personalized advice tailored to your specific health situation, ensuring that the dietary changes you make are safe and beneficial for you.

Additionally, please be aware that the nutritional information provided with each recipe is approximate. Variations in ingredients, brands, and preparation methods can lead to differences in the nutritional content of your meals. While we've done our best to provide accurate information, the exact values may vary. Always consider these approximations as helpful guidelines rather than exact figures.

Furthermore, If our cookbook has brought joy to your kitchen and table, we'd be thrilled to hear about your experiences in an Amazon review. On the flip side, if you stumble upon any hiccups while exploring our recipes, don't hesitate to get in touch at **kloppkingsley@gmail.com.** We're here to support your cooking journey every step of the way.

We hope this cookbook becomes a valuable tool in your journey towards managing CRPS and improving your quality of life. Our goal is to offer you tasty, nourishing options that bring joy to your meals and support your health. Remember, you are the best expert on your own body, so listen to it, experiment with the recipes, and find what works best for you.

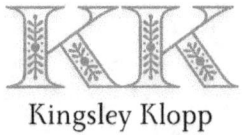

Kingsley Klopp

Introduction.

Welcome to the **Complex Regional Pain Syndrome (CRPS) Diet Cookbook for Beginners!** If you've picked up this book, chances are you're navigating the challenging waters of CRPS, and you're looking for ways to ease your symptoms through the power of nutrition. You're in the right place. We're about to embark on a culinary journey that not only aims to tantalize your taste buds but also help you manage your pain and improve your overall well-being. Let's be honest: living with CRPS is tough. The constant pain, the unpredictability, and the way it can disrupt your daily life can be overwhelming. But here's the good news: what you eat can make a difference. And no, we're not talking about bland, boring meals that leave you unsatisfied. We're talking about delicious, nutritious dishes that you'll actually look forward to eating. Imagine waking up and looking forward to a breakfast that doesn't just fill you up but also helps in reducing inflammation and alleviating pain. Picture yourself preparing a dinner that's not only a feast for your eyes but also packed with ingredients that support your healing process. This cookbook is designed with you in mind. We know that managing CRPS involves a lot of trial and error, and sometimes it feels like you're constantly searching for something that works. That's why we've compiled recipes that are easy to follow, made with accessible ingredients, and specifically chosen for their anti-inflammatory and pain-relief properties. But more than that, we've crafted this book to be your companion in the kitchen, guiding you with tips, tricks, and little nuggets of wisdom to make cooking enjoyable and stress-free.

One of the key principles behind our recipes is the emphasis on whole, unprocessed foods. You'll find an abundance of fruits, vegetables, lean proteins, and healthy fats that not only nourish your body but also help combat inflammation. Think vibrant salads bursting with color and flavor, hearty soups that warm your soul, and delectable desserts that you can indulge in without guilt. We believe that food should be a source of joy and comfort, not just a necessity, and we've infused that philosophy into every page of this cookbook. But this book is more than just a collection of recipes. It's a call to embrace a new way of eating, one that aligns with your body's needs and helps you regain control over your health. Each recipe comes with detailed instructions, nutritional information, and tips on how to make the most out of your meals.

We've also included sections on understanding CRPS, the role of diet in managing symptoms, and practical advice on shopping and meal planning. So, let's get started. Grab your apron, head to the kitchen, and let's cook up some delicious, healing meals together. Whether you're a seasoned cook or a complete novice, this cookbook is here to support you every step of the way. Let's turn the page on pain and start a new chapter of wellness and delicious dining. Welcome to the **Complex Regional Pain Syndrome (CRPS) Diet Cookbook for Beginners** – your new culinary adventure awaits!

Chapter 1: The Basics of CRPS and Nutrition

What is Complex Regional Pain Syndrome (CRPS)?

Complex Regional Pain Syndrome (CRPS) is a chronic, often debilitating condition characterized by severe, persistent pain that usually affects an arm, leg, hand, or foot. The pain associated with CRPS is far more intense and prolonged than what would be expected from the initial injury. This condition not only challenges the physical endurance of those afflicted but also takes a substantial toll on their emotional and mental well-being.

A Brief History of CRPS

The history of CRPS dates back to the American Civil War when it was first identified by a Confederate doctor, Dr. Silas Weir Mitchell, who coined the term "causalgia" to describe the intense, burning pain experienced by soldiers after limb injuries. Over time, the understanding of this condition evolved, and it was recognized that similar pain could develop after relatively minor injuries as well. In 1994, the International Association for the Study of Pain (IASP) introduced the term Complex Regional Pain Syndrome to encompass a broader range of symptoms and causes.

The Evolution of Understanding

CRPS has undergone significant changes in understanding and classification over the years. Initially, it was thought to be primarily a nerve injury, but further research revealed a more complex interplay of the nervous, immune, and vascular systems. This understanding has led to the classification of CRPS into two main types:

- CRPS Type I: Previously known as Reflex Sympathetic Dystrophy (RSD), this type occurs without a confirmed nerve injury. It is the more common form and can develop after a minor injury, such as a sprain or fracture.
- CRPS Type II: Formerly called causalgia, this type is associated with a distinct nerve injury. It is less common but can be more severe and challenging to treat.

The Mechanisms Behind CRPS

The exact cause of CRPS remains elusive, but it is generally believed to involve a combination of factors, including:

1. Abnormal Pain Signal Processing: In CRPS, the nervous system amplifies pain signals in response to injury, causing severe pain that persists long after the injury has healed.

2. Inflammatory Responses: The immune system may react excessively to the injury, releasing inflammatory substances that contribute to pain and swelling.

3. Vascular Abnormalities: Changes in blood flow and abnormal dilation or constriction of blood vessels can lead to temperature changes and discoloration in the affected limb.

4. Central Sensitization: The brain and spinal cord may become hypersensitive to pain signals, leading to an exaggerated pain response.

The Emotional and Psychological Impact

Living with CRPS is a daily battle. The unrelenting pain can make even the simplest tasks seem insurmountable. Many individuals with CRPS experience significant emotional distress, including anxiety, depression, and feelings of isolation. The uncertainty of flare-ups and the fear of worsening symptoms can make planning for the future seem daunting.

Treatment and Management

Despite the challenges, there is hope for those living with CRPS. Treatment is often multidisciplinary, involving pain specialists, physical therapists, psychologists, and occupational therapists. The goal is to manage pain, improve function, and enhance quality of life. Common treatments include:

- Medications: Pain relievers, anti-inflammatory drugs, and medications targeting nerve pain can provide some relief.
- Physical Therapy: Gentle, graded exercises help maintain mobility and reduce pain.
- Psychological Support: Cognitive-behavioral therapy (CBT) and other therapeutic approaches can help manage the emotional impact of CRPS.
- Interventional Procedures: Nerve blocks, spinal cord stimulation, and other invasive techniques may be considered in severe cases.
- Alternative Therapies: Techniques such as acupuncture, biofeedback, and mirror therapy have shown promise in some individuals.

The Path Forward

Awareness and education about CRPS are crucial in advancing understanding and improving care. Researchers are continuously exploring new avenues for treatment, including novel medications and innovative approaches to pain management. Support networks and advocacy groups play a vital role in providing resources, raising awareness, and fostering a sense of community among those affected by CRPS.

Symptoms and Triggers

Symptoms of CRPS

1. Chronic Pain
The hallmark symptom of CRPS is persistent, severe pain that can be described as burning, throbbing, or stabbing. This pain often exceeds what would be expected from the initial injury and can spread to other parts of the body.

2. Sensory Disturbances
Individuals with CRPS often experience heightened sensitivity to touch (allodynia), where even light contact can provoke significant pain. Hyperalgesia, an increased sensitivity to pain, is also common.

3. Temperature Changes
Affected areas may feel unusually warm or cold compared to the rest of the body. These temperature changes can fluctuate and are often accompanied by color changes in the skin, ranging from red to blue or purple.

4. Swelling and Edema
Swelling in the affected limb is a frequent symptom, sometimes severe enough to cause significant discomfort and restricted movement.

5. Skin and Nail Changes
The skin over the affected area may become thin, shiny, or excessively sweaty. Changes in nail growth, such as accelerated or slowed growth and brittle nails, are also common.

6. Joint Stiffness and Muscle Weakness
CRPS can lead to joint stiffness, reduced range of motion, and muscle weakness. Over time, this can result in atrophy of the muscles and a decrease in the functionality of the affected limb.

7. Motor Dysfunction
Involuntary muscle spasms, tremors, and dystonia (abnormal muscle tone) can occur. These motor disturbances can significantly impact daily activities and quality of life.

8. Bone and Tissue Changes
Long-term CRPS can lead to changes in bone density (osteopenia or osteoporosis) and soft tissue abnormalities. This can increase the risk of fractures and other complications.

9. Emotional and Psychological Symptoms
Living with chronic pain can lead to anxiety, depression, and a decreased overall sense of well-being. The unpredictability of CRPS symptoms can contribute to emotional distress and social isolation.

Triggers of CRPS

1. Physical Injuries

CRPS often develops after an injury, such as a fracture, sprain, or surgery. These injuries can set off a disproportionate response from the nervous system, leading to the development of CRPS.

2. Surgery

Post-surgical complications, including prolonged immobilization and nerve damage, can trigger CRPS. The body's response to surgical trauma may include abnormal inflammation and pain signaling.

3. Minor Trauma

Even seemingly minor injuries, such as a small cut or bruise, can trigger CRPS in susceptible individuals. The body's exaggerated response to these minor traumas can lead to the syndrome's onset.

4. Immobilization

Prolonged immobilization of a limb, such as wearing a cast or splint for an extended period, can trigger CRPS. The lack of movement can exacerbate abnormal pain signaling and inflammation.

5. Emotional Stress

Stress and emotional trauma can exacerbate CRPS symptoms. The connection between the nervous system and stress responses can amplify pain and other symptoms, making stress management a crucial aspect of CRPS care.

6. Infections

Infections that affect the nerves or tissues in the affected area can trigger CRPS. The immune system's response to infection may include inflammation and altered pain perception.

7. Weather Changes

Some individuals with CRPS report that changes in weather, particularly cold and damp conditions, can exacerbate their symptoms. These changes may affect blood flow and nerve function.

Managing Symptoms and Avoiding Triggers

Managing CRPS involves a comprehensive approach that addresses both symptoms and potential triggers. Here are some strategies that can help:

1. Medication

Pain relief can be achieved through various medications, including anti-inflammatory drugs, nerve pain medications, and corticosteroids. Each individual's treatment plan should be tailored to their specific needs.

2. Physical Therapy

Regular, gentle physical therapy can help maintain joint mobility, reduce stiffness, and improve overall function. It's important to work with a therapist experienced in CRPS to avoid exacerbating symptoms.

3. Psychological Support

Cognitive-behavioral therapy (CBT) and other forms of psychological support can help manage the emotional impact of CRPS. Techniques for stress management and coping skills are essential components of treatment.

4. Lifestyle Modifications

Adopting a healthy lifestyle, including a balanced diet, regular exercise, and adequate sleep, can support overall well-being and potentially reduce the severity of symptoms.

5. Avoiding Known Triggers

Identifying and avoiding known triggers, such as certain physical activities, stressful situations, or extreme weather conditions, can help manage CRPS. Keeping a symptom diary can be useful in recognizing patterns and triggers.

The Importance of Nutrition in CRPS Management

The Healing Power of Food

Food is more than just sustenance; it is a source of healing and strength. For individuals with CRPS, nutrition plays a vital role in modulating pain, reducing inflammation, and supporting overall health. By making mindful dietary choices, those suffering from CRPS can take control of one aspect of their health, empowering themselves to face each day with greater resilience.

Reducing Inflammation Through Diet

Inflammation is a significant component of CRPS, contributing to pain and other debilitating symptoms. An anti-inflammatory diet can help mitigate these effects and provide much-needed relief. Foods rich in omega-3 fatty acids, such as salmon, flaxseeds, and walnuts, have potent anti-inflammatory properties. Including these foods in the diet can help reduce the inflammatory processes that exacerbate CRPS symptoms.

Antioxidant-rich fruits and vegetables, like berries, leafy greens, and colorful vegetables, also play a crucial role in fighting inflammation. These foods are packed with vitamins, minerals, and phytonutrients that protect the body from oxidative stress and promote healing. Embracing a diet rich in these natural powerhouses can make a tangible difference in managing CRPS.

Supporting Nervous System Health

CRPS affects the nervous system, leading to abnormal pain signals and sensory disturbances. Nutrients that support nerve health are essential for individuals with CRPS. Vitamin B12, found in foods like eggs, dairy, and fortified cereals, is crucial for maintaining healthy nerve function. Similarly, magnesium, present in leafy greens, nuts, and whole grains, supports nerve transmission and can alleviate muscle cramps and spasms associated with CRPS. By nourishing the nervous system with these vital nutrients, individuals with CRPS can help stabilize their symptoms and enhance their overall neurological health. This dietary approach offers a proactive way to address the underlying issues that contribute to their pain and discomfort.

Promoting Emotional Well-being

Living with chronic pain can take a significant toll on mental health. Feelings of anxiety, depression, and isolation are common among those with CRPS. Nutrition can play a supportive role in mental well-being, providing the brain with the necessary building blocks to function optimally. Foods rich in omega-3 fatty acids, such as fatty fish, chia seeds, and hemp seeds, have been shown to improve mood and cognitive function. Additionally, foods containing tryptophan, an amino acid found in turkey, cheese, and nuts, can boost serotonin levels, enhancing mood and promoting a sense of calm. A balanced diet that includes these mood-boosting foods can help individuals with CRPS manage the emotional challenges that accompany chronic pain, fostering a more positive outlook and better mental health.

Hydration: The Unsung Hero

Adequate hydration is often overlooked but is crucial for managing CRPS. Dehydration can exacerbate pain and inflammation, making symptoms more difficult to manage. Drinking enough water throughout the day helps maintain proper bodily functions, supports joint lubrication, and aids in nutrient absorption. Herbal teas and water-rich foods like cucumbers, melons, and citrus fruits can contribute to overall hydration. Staying well-hydrated is a simple yet powerful way to support the body's healing processes and reduce the severity of CRPS symptoms.

Key Nutrients for CRPS Patients

Omega-3 Fatty Acids

Why They Matter: Omega-3 fatty acids are renowned for their powerful anti-inflammatory properties. They help reduce the inflammatory response that exacerbates CRPS symptoms, thereby alleviating pain and swelling.

Sources:

- Fatty fish (salmon, mackerel, sardines)
- Flaxseeds and flaxseed oil
- Chia seeds
- Walnuts
- Hemp seeds

Incorporation Tips: Including fatty fish in your diet a few times a week can significantly boost your intake of omega-3s. For vegetarians or those who prefer plant-based options, adding chia seeds or flaxseeds to smoothies, oatmeal, or salads is an easy way to incorporate these beneficial fats.

Magnesium

Why It Matters: Magnesium plays a vital role in nerve function, muscle relaxation, and reducing muscle cramps and spasms often associated with CRPS. It also supports overall nervous system health, which is crucial for managing the condition.

Sources:

- Leafy green vegetables (spinach, kale)
- Nuts and seeds (almonds, sunflower seeds)
- Whole grains (brown rice, quinoa)
- Legumes (black beans, lentils)
- Avocados

Incorporation Tips: Consuming a variety of magnesium-rich foods daily can help ensure adequate intake. For example, start your day with a smoothie containing spinach and avocado, snack on a handful of almonds, and include a serving of quinoa in your lunch or dinner.

Vitamin B12

Why It Matters: Vitamin B12 is essential for maintaining healthy nerve cells and producing DNA. A deficiency in B12 can lead to nerve damage and exacerbate the symptoms of CRPS.

Sources:

- Animal products (meat, poultry, fish)
- Dairy products (milk, cheese, yogurt)
- Eggs
- Fortified cereals and plant-based milks

Incorporation Tips: Including animal products in your diet is an excellent way to ensure sufficient B12 intake. For those following a vegetarian or vegan diet, fortified foods or B12 supplements may be necessary to meet daily requirements.

Antioxidants

Why They Matter: Antioxidants help protect the body from oxidative stress and inflammation, both of which are significant factors in CRPS. They neutralize free radicals, reducing damage to cells and tissues.

Sources:
- Berries (blueberries, strawberries, raspberries)
- Dark chocolate
- Pecans
- Artichokes
- Spinach and kale

Incorporation Tips: Adding a variety of colorful fruits and vegetables to your meals ensures a robust intake of antioxidants. Berries can be enjoyed fresh, in smoothies, or as a topping for yogurt and cereal. Dark chocolate, in moderation, can be a delightful and beneficial treat.

Vitamin D

Why It Matters: Vitamin D is crucial for bone health and immune function. It helps reduce inflammation and supports the nervous system, both of which are important for managing CRPS.

Sources:
- Sunlight exposure
- Fatty fish (salmon, mackerel, sardines)
- Fortified foods (milk, orange juice, cereals)
- Egg yolks

Incorporation Tips: Spending a few minutes in the sun each day can boost your Vitamin D levels. Additionally, including fatty fish and fortified foods in your diet helps ensure adequate intake. In some cases, supplements may be necessary, especially during the winter months or for those with limited sun exposure.

Zinc

Why It Matters: Zinc plays a role in immune function and wound healing. It also helps reduce inflammation and supports overall health, which can be beneficial for CRPS patients.

Sources:
- Meat and poultry
- Shellfish (oysters, crab, lobster)
- Legumes (chickpeas, lentils)
- Seeds (pumpkin, sesame)
- Nuts (cashews, almonds)

Incorporation Tips: Including a variety of zinc-rich foods in your diet helps meet your daily needs. Enjoy shellfish as a part of your regular meal rotation, and snack on nuts and seeds to boost your zinc intake.

Probiotics

Why They Matter: Probiotics are beneficial bacteria that support gut health. A healthy gut can help reduce inflammation and improve immune function, both of which are important for managing CRPS symptoms.

Sources:

- Yogurt with live cultures
- Kefir
- Sauerkraut
- Kimchi
- Kombucha

Incorporation Tips: Incorporating probiotic-rich foods into your diet can support gut health and reduce inflammation. Enjoy a serving of yogurt or kefir with your breakfast, or add sauerkraut or kimchi to your meals.

Anti-Inflammatory Diet Principles

An anti-inflammatory diet is not just a regimen; it's a lifestyle that promotes overall well-being by reducing inflammation in the body. For individuals suffering from chronic conditions like Complex Regional Pain Syndrome (CRPS), embracing these dietary principles can be a game-changer. Inflammation is a key driver of pain and other symptoms in CRPS, making an anti-inflammatory diet an essential component of managing the condition effectively.

The Foundation of an Anti-Inflammatory Diet
The core idea behind an anti-inflammatory diet is to focus on foods that help reduce inflammation and avoid those that can trigger or exacerbate it. This approach is not just beneficial for those with CRPS but also for anyone looking to improve their overall health and prevent chronic diseases.
Key Principles of an Anti-Inflammatory Diet
1. Emphasize Whole Foods
Why It Matters: Whole foods are minimally processed and retain their natural nutrients, which are essential for reducing inflammation. They are free from additives, preservatives, and refined sugars that can contribute to inflammation.
Examples:
- Fresh fruits and vegetables
- Whole grains (quinoa, brown rice, oats)
- Lean proteins (chicken, fish, legumes)
- Nuts and seeds

Incorporation Tips: Fill your plate with a variety of colorful fruits and vegetables, aim for whole grains over refined ones, and choose lean proteins. Snacking on nuts and seeds can also help maintain a balanced diet.
2. Prioritize Omega-3 Fatty Acids
Why It Matters: Omega-3 fatty acids have strong anti-inflammatory properties and play a crucial role in reducing chronic inflammation. They also support heart and brain health.
Sources:
- Fatty fish (salmon, mackerel, sardines)
- Flaxseeds and flaxseed oil
- Chia seeds
- Walnuts

Incorporation Tips: Include fatty fish in your diet at least twice a week. Add flaxseeds or chia seeds to your smoothies, yogurt, or oatmeal. Walnuts make for a great snack or salad topping.

3. Consume Antioxidant-Rich Foods

Why It Matters: Antioxidants protect the body from oxidative stress, which can trigger inflammation. They neutralize free radicals and reduce damage to cells and tissues.

Sources:

- Berries (blueberries, strawberries, raspberries)
- Dark leafy greens (spinach, kale)
- Nuts and seeds
- Dark chocolate (in moderation)

Incorporation Tips: Enjoy a variety of berries as snacks or in your breakfast. Include dark leafy greens in salads, smoothies, or as a side dish. Treat yourself to a small piece of dark chocolate for dessert.

4. Choose Healthy Fats

Why It Matters: Healthy fats, such as monounsaturated and polyunsaturated fats, help reduce inflammation and support overall health. Avoid trans fats and excessive saturated fats, which can increase inflammation.

Sources:

- Olive oil
- Avocados
- Nuts and seeds
- Fatty fish

Incorporation Tips: Use olive oil as your primary cooking oil and for salad dressings. Add avocado to your sandwiches, salads, or smoothies. Nuts and seeds are excellent for snacking and cooking.

5. Limit Refined Carbohydrates and Sugars

Why It Matters: Refined carbohydrates and sugars can spike blood sugar levels and promote inflammation. They are often found in processed foods, which lack essential nutrients.

Sources to Avoid:

- White bread and pastries
- Sugary beverages
- Candy and sweets
- Processed snack foods

Incorporation Tips: Opt for whole grain alternatives like brown rice, quinoa, and whole-wheat bread. Replace sugary snacks with fruits and nuts. Choose water, herbal teas, or natural fruit juices over sugary drinks.

6. Include Herbs and Spices

Why It Matters: Many herbs and spices have anti-inflammatory properties and can enhance the flavor of your meals without added sodium or unhealthy fats.

Examples:

- Turmeric
- Ginger
- Garlic
- Cinnamon

Incorporation Tips: Incorporate these herbs and spices into your cooking. For example, add turmeric and ginger to soups and stews, garlic to sauces and dressings, and cinnamon to oatmeal or smoothies.

The Benefits of an Anti-Inflammatory Diet

Adopting an anti-inflammatory diet can offer numerous benefits, particularly for those with CRPS:

- Reduced Pain and Inflammation: By focusing on anti-inflammatory foods, individuals can help decrease the overall level of inflammation in their bodies, leading to reduced pain and discomfort.
- Improved Immune Function: A balanced diet rich in whole foods, antioxidants, and healthy fats supports a healthy immune system, which is crucial for managing chronic conditions.
- Enhanced Energy Levels: Nutrient-dense foods provide sustained energy, helping to combat the fatigue often associated with chronic pain.
- Better Mental Health: Proper nutrition can improve mood and cognitive function, offering emotional support for those dealing with the psychological impacts of CRPS.

Foods to Avoid for CRPS Patients

Complex Regional Pain Syndrome (CRPS) is a challenging condition characterized by severe, persistent pain and a host of other debilitating symptoms. While an anti-inflammatory diet can play a crucial role in managing CRPS, it is equally important to avoid certain foods that can exacerbate inflammation and worsen symptoms. Below is a comprehensive guide to the foods that CRPS patients should avoid to help manage their condition effectively.

Refined Carbohydrates

Why to Avoid: Refined carbohydrates can cause spikes in blood sugar levels, leading to increased inflammation. They lack essential nutrients and fiber, which can contribute to weight gain and other health issues that may aggravate CRPS symptoms.

Examples:
- White bread
- Pastries
- White rice
- Sugary cereals
- Pasta made from refined flour

Alternatives: Opt for whole grain alternatives such as brown rice, quinoa, whole-wheat bread, and whole-grain pasta, which provide more nutrients and fiber.

Sugary Foods and Beverages

Why to Avoid: High sugar intake is linked to increased inflammation and can worsen pain and other symptoms in CRPS patients. Sugary foods and drinks can also lead to weight gain, which puts additional strain on the body.

Examples:
- Sodas and sugary drinks
- Candy and sweets
- Baked goods with high sugar content
- Ice cream and desserts
- Processed snacks

Alternatives: Choose natural sweeteners like honey or maple syrup in moderation, and enjoy fresh fruits as a healthier option for satisfying sweet cravings. Drink water, herbal teas, or naturally flavored water instead of sugary beverages.

Trans Fats

Why to Avoid: Trans fats are known to increase inflammation and contribute to various chronic diseases. They are found in many processed and fried foods and can exacerbate CRPS symptoms.

Examples:

- Margarine and shortening
- Commercially baked goods (cookies, cakes, pies)
- **Fried fast foods**
- Snack foods (chips, microwave popcorn)
- Processed and packaged foods

Alternatives: Use healthy fats like olive oil, avocado oil, or coconut oil for cooking. Choose baked or grilled foods instead of fried options.

Excessive Saturated Fats

Why to Avoid: While some saturated fats can be part of a healthy diet, excessive intake can lead to increased inflammation and other health issues. Saturated fats are typically found in animal products and certain oils.

Examples:

- Fatty cuts of meat (beef, pork)
- Processed meats (sausages, bacon)
- Full-fat dairy products (butter, cream, cheese)
- Palm oil and coconut oil (in large quantities)

Alternatives: Opt for lean cuts of meat, skinless poultry, and low-fat or non-dairy alternatives. Incorporate more plant-based proteins and healthy fats into your diet.

Artificial Additives and Preservatives

Why to Avoid: Artificial additives and preservatives can trigger inflammation and other adverse reactions in some individuals. They are commonly found in processed and packaged foods.

Examples:

- Artificial sweeteners (aspartame, saccharin)
- Food colorings
- Flavor enhancers (MSG)
- Preservatives (sodium benzoate, nitrates)
- Packaged snacks and ready-to-eat meals

Alternatives: Choose whole, unprocessed foods whenever possible. Read labels carefully and avoid products with long lists of additives and preservatives.

Alcohol

Why to Avoid: Excessive alcohol consumption can lead to increased inflammation and exacerbate CRPS symptoms. It can also interfere with medications and other treatments used to manage the condition.

Examples:
- Beer
- Wine
- Spirits
- Cocktails with sugary mixers

Alternatives: If you choose to drink, do so in moderation. Opt for healthier alternatives like sparkling water with a splash of natural juice or herbal teas.

Caffeine

Why to Avoid: While moderate caffeine intake may not be harmful to everyone, excessive consumption can lead to increased stress and inflammation. It can also interfere with sleep, which is crucial for managing CRPS symptoms.

Examples:
- Coffee (in large quantities)
- Energy drinks
- High-caffeine teas
- Soft drinks with caffeine

Alternatives: Limit caffeine intake to moderate levels and choose caffeine-free alternatives like herbal teas, decaffeinated coffee, or water.

High-Sodium Foods

Why to Avoid: High sodium intake can lead to fluid retention and increased blood pressure, which can exacerbate CRPS symptoms. Processed and packaged foods are often high in sodium.

Examples:
- Processed meats (ham, bacon, sausages)
- Canned soups and vegetables
- Packaged snacks (chips, crackers)
- Fast foods
- Frozen meals

Alternatives: Use herbs and spices to flavor your food instead of salt. Choose fresh, whole foods and prepare meals at home to control sodium intake.

Nightshade Vegetables (for some individuals)

Why to Avoid: Nightshade vegetables contain solanine, which can cause inflammation and pain in some individuals. This group of vegetables may exacerbate CRPS symptoms in sensitive individuals.

Examples:
- Tomatoes
- Potatoes
- Eggplants
- Peppers (bell peppers, chili peppers)

Alternatives: If you suspect nightshades are contributing to your symptoms, try eliminating them and replacing them with other vegetables like leafy greens, carrots, and squash. Consult with a healthcare provider or nutritionist before making significant dietary changes.

Breakfast Recipes

1. Oatmeal with Chopped Apples and Cinnamon
Ingredients:
- 1 cup rolled oats
- 2 cups water or almond milk
- 1 medium apple, chopped
- 1 teaspoon ground cinnamon
- 1 tablespoon chia seeds
- 1 tablespoon maple syrup (optional)
- 1/4 teaspoon vanilla extract
- 1/4 cup chopped walnuts

Instructions:
1. In a medium saucepan, bring the water or almond milk to a boil.
2. Add the rolled oats and reduce the heat to a simmer. Cook for about 5 minutes, stirring occasionally.
3. Stir in the chopped apple, ground cinnamon, chia seeds, and vanilla extract. Continue to cook for another 2-3 minutes, until the oats are tender and the apple pieces are soft.
4. Remove from heat and stir in the maple syrup, if using.
5. Serve topped with chopped walnuts.

Nutrition Info per Serving (Serves 2):
- Calories: 300
- Protein: 7g
- Carbohydrates: 50g
- Fiber: 8g
- Sugars: 12g
- Fat: 10g
- Saturated Fat: 1g

Cooking Time:
- **Total: 10 minutes**

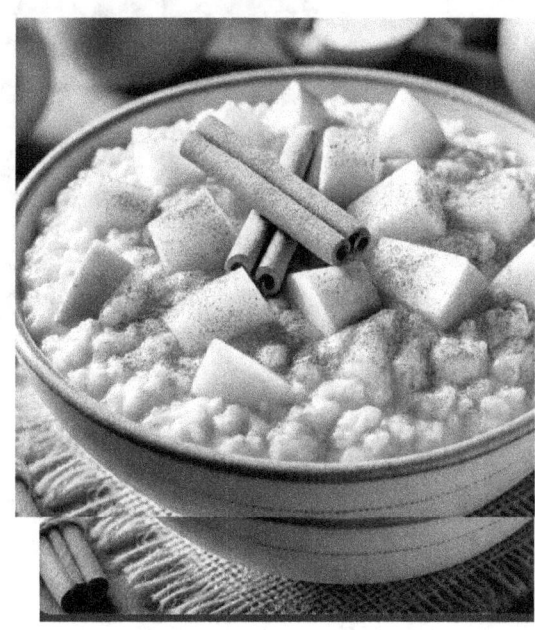

2. Smoothie Bowl with Berries and Seeds

Ingredients:

- 1 banana, frozen
- 1/2 cup frozen mixed berries (strawberries, blueberries, raspberries)
- 1/2 cup unsweetened almond milk
- 1 tablespoon chia seeds
- 1 tablespoon flaxseeds
- 1 tablespoon almond butter
- 1/4 cup granola (sugar-free)
- Fresh berries and sliced almonds for topping

Instructions:

1. In a blender, combine the frozen banana, frozen mixed berries, and almond milk. Blend until smooth.
2. Pour the smoothie into a bowl.
3. Top with chia seeds, flaxseeds, almond butter, granola, fresh berries, and sliced almonds.
4. Serve immediately.

Nutrition Info per Serving (Serves 1):

- Calories: 400
- Protein: 10g
- Carbohydrates: 55g
- Fiber: 12g
- Sugars: 20g
- Fat: 18g
- Saturated Fat: 2g

Cooking Time:

- **Total: 5 minutes**

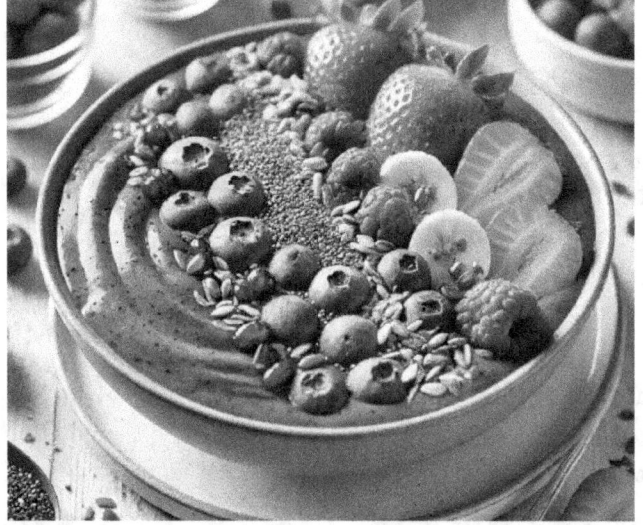

3. Buckwheat Pancakes

Ingredients:

- 1 cup buckwheat flour
- 1 tablespoon baking powder
- 1/2 teaspoon ground cinnamon
- 1 cup almond milk
- 1 tablespoon maple syrup
- 1 teaspoon vanilla extract
- 1 egg, beaten
- Coconut oil for cooking

Instructions:

1. In a large bowl, whisk together the buckwheat flour, baking powder, and ground cinnamon.
2. In another bowl, mix the almond milk, maple syrup, vanilla extract, and beaten egg.
3. Pour the wet ingredients into the dry ingredients and stir until just combined.
4. Heat a small amount of coconut oil in a non-stick skillet over medium heat.
5. Pour 1/4 cup of batter onto the skillet for each pancake. Cook until bubbles form on the surface, then flip and cook until browned on the other side.
6. Repeat with the remaining batter, adding more coconut oil as needed.
7. Serve warm with fresh fruit or a drizzle of maple syrup.

Nutrition Info per Serving (Serves 4):

- Calories: 180
- Protein: 5g
- Carbohydrates: 25g
- Fiber: 4g
- Sugars: 5g
- Fat: 6g
- Saturated Fat: 3g

Cooking Time:

- **Total: 20 minutes**

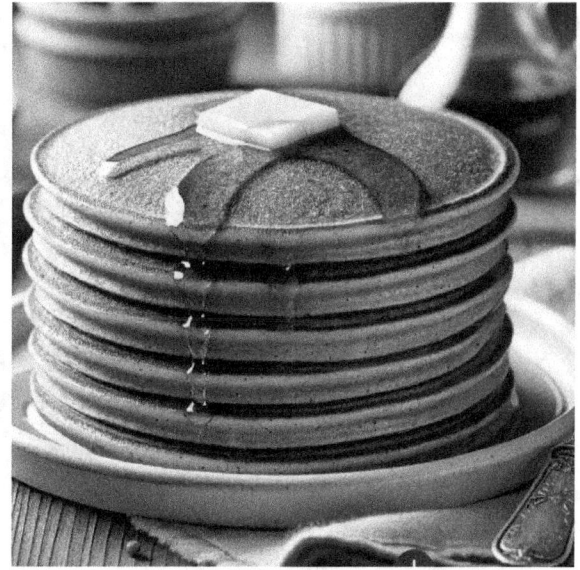

4. Sweet Potato Hash

Ingredients:

- 2 medium sweet potatoes, peeled and diced
- 1 red bell pepper, diced
- 1 green bell pepper, diced
- 1 small onion, diced
- 2 tablespoons olive oil
- 1 teaspoon ground cumin
- 1/2 teaspoon smoked paprika
- 1/4 teaspoon turmeric
- Fresh parsley for garnish

Instructions:

1. Heat the olive oil in a large skillet over medium heat.
2. Add the diced sweet potatoes, red bell pepper, green bell pepper, and onion to the skillet. Cook for 10-15 minutes, stirring occasionally, until the vegetables are tender.
3. Stir in the ground cumin, smoked paprika, and turmeric. Cook for an additional 2-3 minutes.
4. Remove from heat and garnish with fresh parsley before serving.

Nutrition Info per Serving (Serves 4):

- Calories: 160
- Protein: 2g
- Carbohydrates: 25g
- Fiber: 5g
- Sugars: 7g
- Fat: 7g
- Saturated Fat: 1g

Cooking Time:

- **Total: 20 minutes**

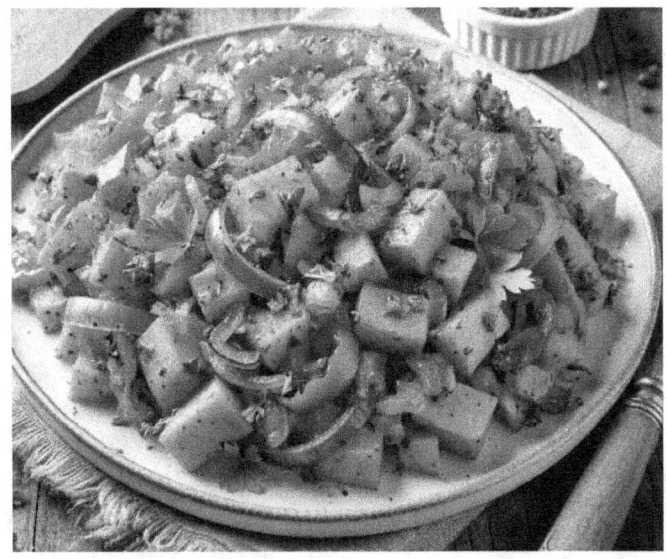

5. Quinoa Porridge

Ingredients:

- 1 cup quinoa, rinsed
- 2 cups almond milk
- 1 teaspoon vanilla extract
- 1 tablespoon maple syrup
- 1/2 teaspoon ground cinnamon
- 1/4 cup chopped nuts (almonds, walnuts)
- Fresh berries for topping

Instructions:

1. In a medium saucepan, combine the rinsed quinoa and almond milk. Bring to a boil.
2. Reduce the heat to low, cover, and simmer for about 15 minutes, or until the quinoa is tender and the liquid is absorbed.
3. Stir in the vanilla extract, maple syrup, and ground cinnamon.
4. Divide the porridge into bowls and top with chopped nuts and fresh berries.
5. Serve warm.

Nutrition Info per Serving (Serves 2):

- Calories: 280
- Protein: 8g
- Carbohydrates: 40g
- Fiber: 5g
- Sugars: 10g
- Fat: 10g
- Saturated Fat: 1g

Cooking Time:

- **Total: 20 minutes**

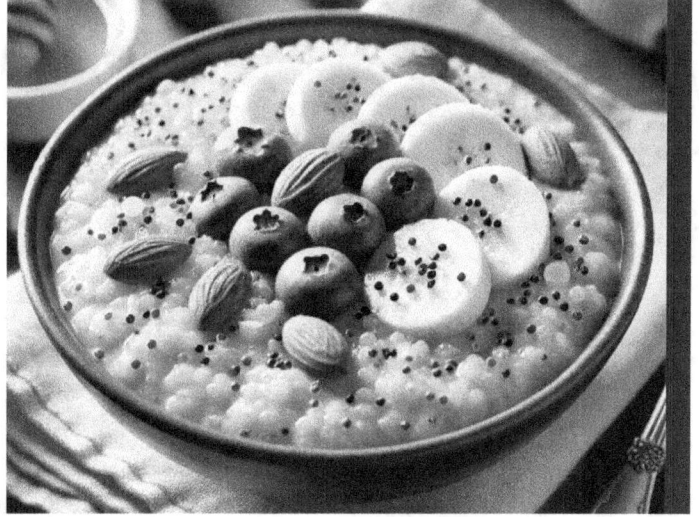

6. Banana Almond Smoothie

Ingredients:

- 1 banana, frozen
- 1 cup unsweetened almond milk
- 2 tablespoons almond butter
- 1 tablespoon chia seeds
- 1/2 teaspoon ground cinnamon
- 1 teaspoon maple syrup (optional)

Instructions:

1. In a blender, combine the frozen banana, almond milk, almond butter, chia seeds, ground cinnamon, and maple syrup (if using).
2. Blend until smooth.
3. Pour into a glass and serve immediately.

Nutrition Info per Serving (Serves 1):

- Calories: 350
- Protein: 7g
- Carbohydrates: 35g
- Fiber: 8g
- Sugars: 16g
- Fat: 20g
- Saturated Fat: 2g

Cooking Time:

- **Total: 5 minutes**

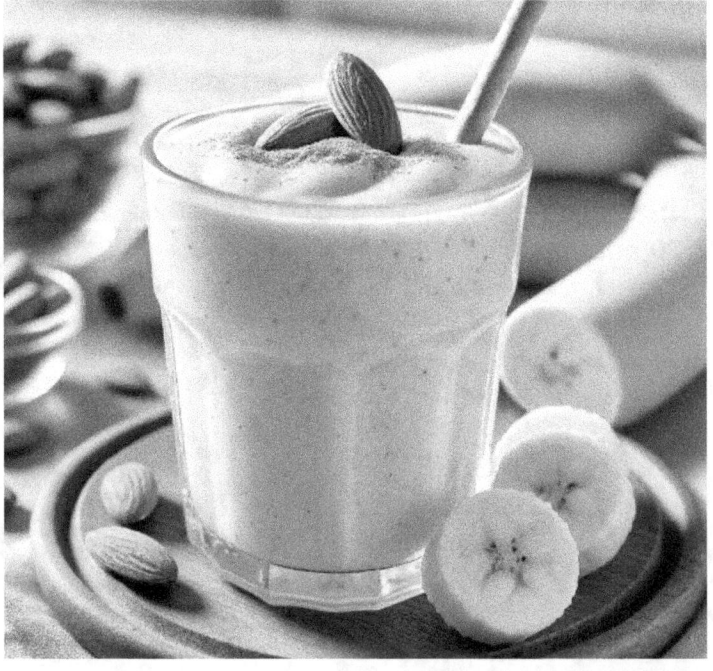

7. Rice Cakes with Almond Butter and Banana Slices

Ingredients:

- 2 whole-grain rice cakes
- 2 tablespoons almond butter
- 1 banana, sliced
- 1 tablespoon chia seeds
- 1 teaspoon honey (optional)

Instructions:

1. Spread 1 tablespoon of almond butter on each rice cake.
2. Top with banana slices.
3. Sprinkle chia seeds over the top.
4. Drizzle with honey, if desired.
5. Serve immediately.

Nutrition Info per Serving (Serves 1):

- Calories: 350
- Protein: 8g
- Carbohydrates: 48g
- Fiber: 8g
- Sugars: 16g
- Fat: 14g
- Saturated Fat: 1.5g

Cooking Time:

- **Total: 5 minutes**

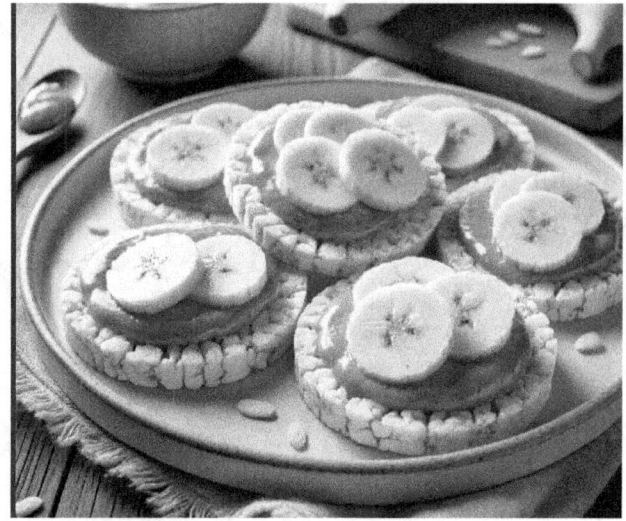

8. Baked Oatmeal Cups

Ingredients:

- 2 cups rolled oats
- 1 teaspoon baking powder
- 1 teaspoon ground cinnamon
- 1/2 teaspoon ground nutmeg
- 2 eggs, beaten
- 1 cup unsweetened almond milk
- 1/4 cup maple syrup
- 1 teaspoon vanilla extract
- 1 cup mixed berries (fresh or frozen)
- 1/4 cup chopped walnuts

Instructions:

1. Preheat the oven to 350°F (175°C).
2. In a large bowl, mix together the rolled oats, baking powder, ground cinnamon, and ground nutmeg.
3. In another bowl, whisk together the eggs, almond milk, maple syrup, and vanilla extract.
4. Combine the wet ingredients with the dry ingredients and mix well.
5. Fold in the mixed berries and chopped walnuts.
6. Divide the mixture evenly among a greased muffin tin (12 cups).
7. Bake for 25-30 minutes, or until the tops are golden and a toothpick inserted into the center comes out clean.
8. Let cool for a few minutes before removing from the muffin tin.
9. Serve warm or store in the refrigerator for up to 5 days.

Nutrition Info per Serving (Serves 12):

- Calories: 120
- Protein: 3g
- Carbohydrates: 18g
- Fiber: 3g
- Sugars: 6g
- Fat: 5g
- Saturated Fat: 0.5g

Cooking Time:

- **Total: 35 minutes**

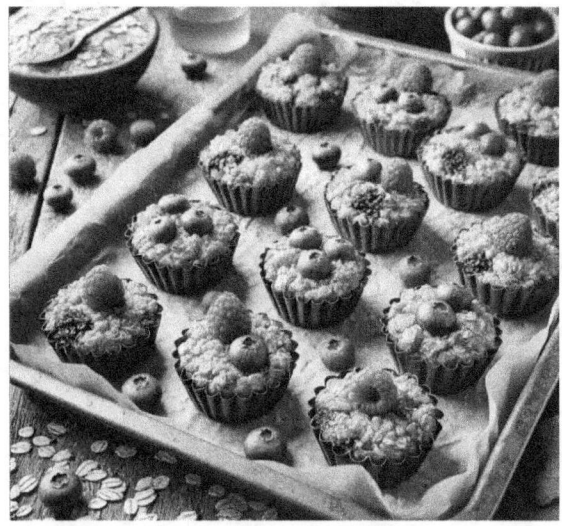

9. Kale and Apple Smoothie

Ingredients:

- 1 cup kale leaves, stems removed
- 1 apple, cored and chopped
- 1 banana, frozen
- 1 cup unsweetened almond milk
- 1 tablespoon flaxseeds
- 1 teaspoon honey (optional)

Instructions:

1. In a blender, combine the kale leaves, chopped apple, frozen banana, almond milk, and flaxseeds.
2. Blend until smooth.
3. Add honey, if desired, and blend again.
4. Pour into a glass and serve immediately.

Nutrition Info per Serving (Serves 1):

- Calories: 250
- Protein: 4g
- Carbohydrates: 50g
- Fiber: 8g
- Sugars: 30g
- Fat: 5g
- Saturated Fat: 0.5g

Cooking Time:

- **Total: 5 minutes**

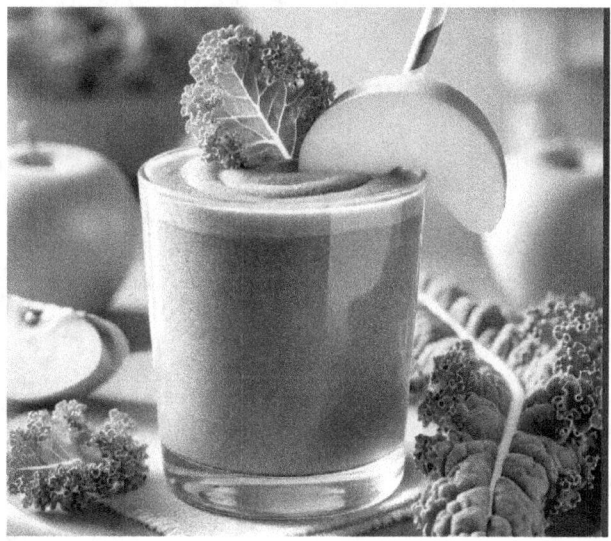

10. Homemade Granola

Ingredients:

- 3 cups rolled oats
- 1 cup nuts (almonds, walnuts, pecans), chopped
- 1/2 cup seeds (pumpkin, sunflower, chia)
- 1/2 cup unsweetened shredded coconut
- 1/4 cup maple syrup
- 1/4 cup coconut oil, melted
- 1 teaspoon vanilla extract
- 1 teaspoon ground cinnamon
- 1/2 cup dried fruit (raisins, cranberries)

Instructions:

1. Preheat the oven to 300°F (150°C).
2. In a large bowl, mix together the rolled oats, chopped nuts, seeds, and shredded coconut.
3. In a small bowl, whisk together the maple syrup, melted coconut oil, vanilla extract, and ground cinnamon.
4. Pour the wet mixture over the dry ingredients and stir until evenly coated.
5. Spread the granola mixture onto a baking sheet lined with parchment paper.
6. Bake for 25-30 minutes, stirring halfway through, until the granola is golden brown.
7. Remove from the oven and let cool completely.
8. Stir in the dried fruit.
9. Store in an airtight container for up to 2 weeks.

Nutrition Info per Serving (Serves 12):

- Calories: 200
- Protein: 4g
- Carbohydrates: 24g
- Fiber: 4g
- Sugars: 8g
- Fat: 11g
- Saturated Fat: 4g

Cooking Time:

- **Total: 35 minutes**

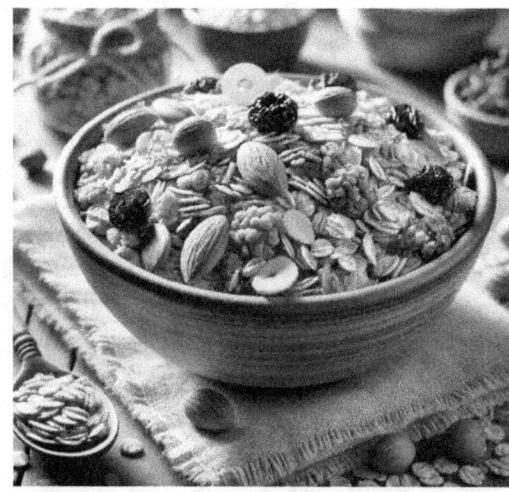

11. Pumpkin Spice Porridge

Ingredients:

- 1 cup rolled oats
- 2 cups unsweetened almond milk
- 1/2 cup pumpkin puree
- 1 teaspoon ground cinnamon
- 1/2 teaspoon ground nutmeg
- 1/4 teaspoon ground ginger
- 1/4 teaspoon ground cloves
- 1 tablespoon maple syrup
- 1/4 cup chopped pecans

Instructions:

1. In a medium saucepan, bring the almond milk to a boil.
2. Stir in the rolled oats, pumpkin puree, cinnamon, nutmeg, ginger, and cloves.
3. Reduce heat to a simmer and cook for 5-7 minutes, stirring occasionally, until the oats are tender and the porridge is thickened.
4. Stir in the maple syrup.
5. Divide into bowls and top with chopped pecans.
6. Serve warm.

Nutrition Info per Serving (Serves 2):

- Calories: 290
- Protein: 6g
- Carbohydrates: 45g
- Fiber: 7g
- Sugars: 12g
- Fat: 10g
- Saturated Fat: 1g

Cooking Time:

- **Total: 10 minutes**

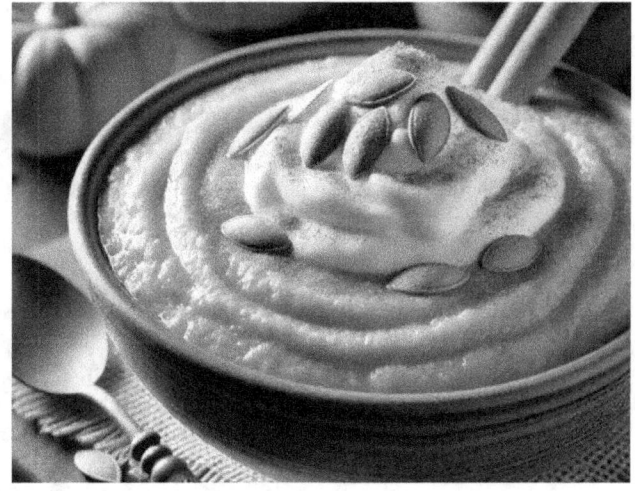

12. Sautéed Vegetables and Quinoa

Ingredients:

- 1 cup quinoa, rinsed
- 2 cups water
- 1 tablespoon olive oil
- 1 small onion, diced
- 1 red bell pepper, diced
- 1 zucchini, diced
- 1 cup cherry tomatoes, halved
- 2 cloves garlic, minced
- 1 teaspoon dried oregano
- 1 teaspoon dried basil
- Fresh parsley for garnish

Instructions:

1. In a medium saucepan, bring water to a boil. Add quinoa, reduce heat to low, cover, and simmer for 15 minutes, or until water is absorbed and quinoa is tender.
2. In a large skillet, heat olive oil over medium heat.
3. Add diced onion and cook for 3-4 minutes, until softened.
4. Add red bell pepper, zucchini, cherry tomatoes, garlic, oregano, and basil. Cook for another 5-7 minutes, until vegetables are tender.
5. Stir in cooked quinoa and mix well.
6. Garnish with fresh parsley and serve warm.

Nutrition Info per Serving (Serves 4):

- Calories: 250
- Protein: 7g
- Carbohydrates: 40g
- Fiber: 6g
- Sugars: 6g
- Fat: 8g
- Saturated Fat: 1g

Cooking Time:

- **Total: 25 minutes**

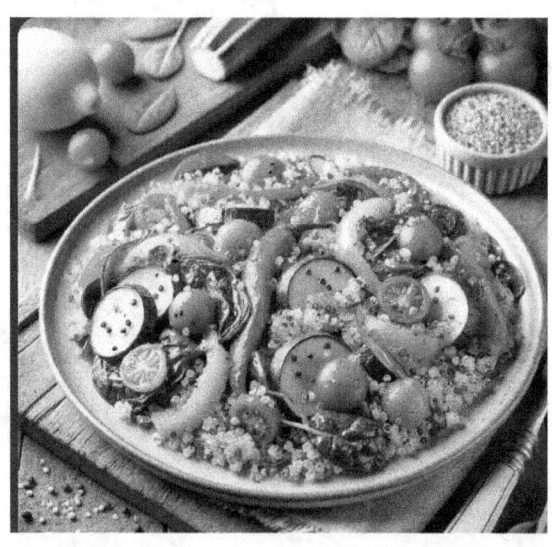

13. Berry and Walnut Salad

Ingredients:

- 4 cups mixed greens (spinach, arugula, kale)
- 1 cup mixed berries (strawberries, blueberries, raspberries)
- 1/4 cup chopped walnuts
- 1/4 cup crumbled feta cheese (optional)
- 2 tablespoons balsamic vinegar
- 2 tablespoons olive oil
- 1 teaspoon honey

Instructions:

1. In a large bowl, combine the mixed greens, mixed berries, chopped walnuts, and feta cheese (if using).
2. In a small bowl, whisk together the balsamic vinegar, olive oil, and honey.
3. Drizzle the dressing over the salad and toss to combine.
4. Serve immediately.

Nutrition Info per Serving (Serves 4):

- Calories: 180
- Protein: 4g
- Carbohydrates: 14g
- Fiber: 4g
- Sugars: 8g
- Fat: 13g
- Saturated Fat: 2g

Cooking Time:

- **Total: 10 minutes**

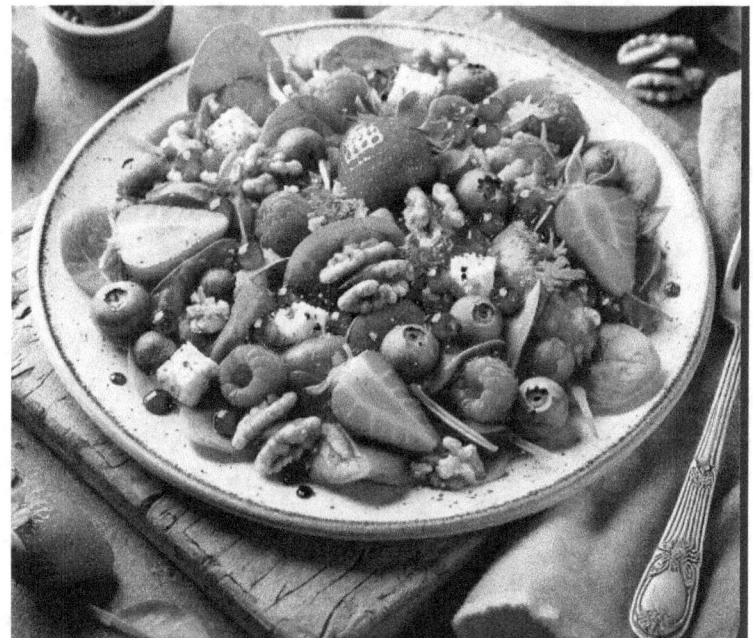

14. Almond Flour Muffins

Ingredients:

- 2 cups almond flour
- 1/4 cup coconut flour
- 1 teaspoon baking soda
- 1/2 teaspoon ground cinnamon
- 1/4 teaspoon ground nutmeg
- 3 eggs
- 1/4 cup maple syrup
- 1/4 cup unsweetened applesauce
- 1 teaspoon vanilla extract
- 1/2 cup blueberries (fresh or frozen)

Instructions:

1. Preheat the oven to 350°F (175°C) and line a muffin tin with paper liners.
2. In a large bowl, mix together the almond flour, coconut flour, baking soda, ground cinnamon, and ground nutmeg.
3. In another bowl, whisk together the eggs, maple syrup, applesauce, and vanilla extract.
4. Pour the wet ingredients into the dry ingredients and stir until just combined.
5. Gently fold in the blueberries.
6. Divide the batter evenly among the muffin cups.
7. Bake for 20-25 minutes, or until a toothpick inserted into the center comes out clean.
8. Let cool in the tin for a few minutes before transferring to a wire rack to cool completely.
9. Serve warm or store in an airtight container for up to 5 days.

Nutrition Info per Serving (Serves 12):

- Calories: 170
- Protein: 5g
- Carbohydrates: 12g
- Fiber: 3g
- Sugars: 7g
- Fat: 12g
- Saturated Fat: 1.5g

Cooking Time:

- **Total: 30 minutes**

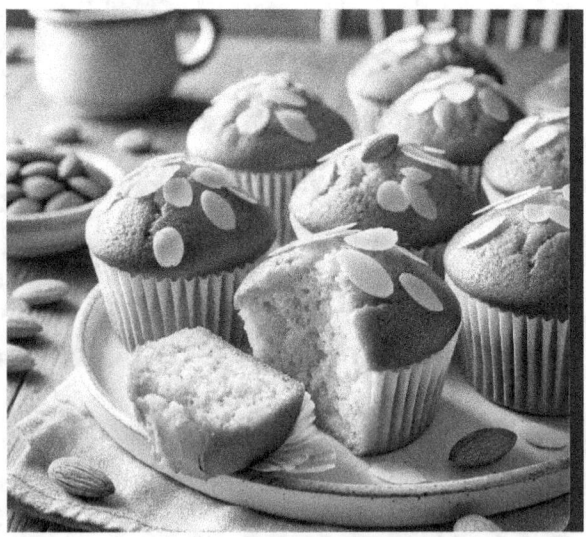

15. Spinach and Mushroom Omelette

Ingredients:

- 2 eggs
- 1/4 cup unsweetened almond milk
- 1 tablespoon olive oil
- 1/2 cup sliced mushrooms
- 1 cup fresh spinach
- 1/4 teaspoon dried thyme
- Fresh chives for garnish

Instructions:

1. In a small bowl, whisk together the eggs and almond milk until well combined.
2. Heat the olive oil in a non-stick skillet over medium heat.
3. Add the sliced mushrooms and cook for 3-4 minutes, until softened.
4. Add the spinach and cook for another 1-2 minutes, until wilted.
5. Pour the egg mixture into the skillet, ensuring it spreads evenly.
6. Sprinkle with dried thyme.
7. Cook for 2-3 minutes, until the edges begin to set, then gently lift the edges with a spatula and tilt the pan to let any uncooked egg flow to the edges.
8. Continue cooking until the omelette is set but still slightly soft in the center.
9. Fold the omelette in half and transfer to a plate.
10. Garnish with fresh chives and serve immediately.

Nutrition Info per Serving (Serves 1):

- Calories: 220
- Protein: 14g
- Carbohydrates: 5g
- Fiber: 2g
- Sugars: 2g
- Fat: 17g
- Saturated Fat: 3.5g

Cooking Time:

- **Total: 10 minutes**

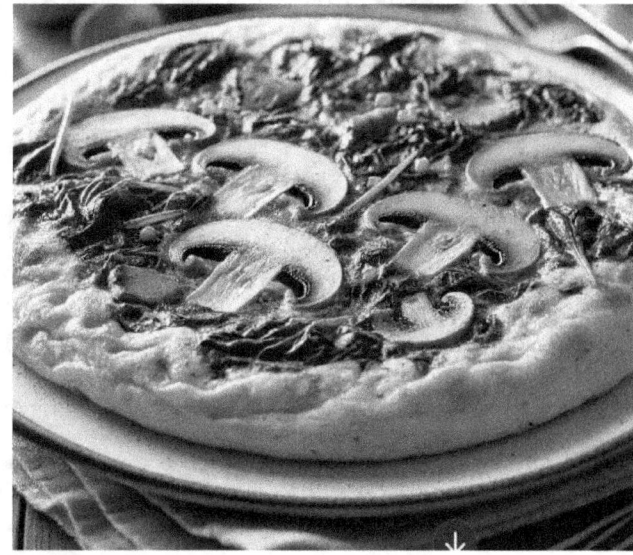

16. Savory Buckwheat Crepes

Ingredients:

- 1 cup buckwheat flour
- 1 1/4 cups water
- 1 egg
- 2 tablespoons olive oil
- 1/2 teaspoon dried thyme
- 1/2 teaspoon dried oregano
- 1 cup fresh spinach
- 1/2 cup cherry tomatoes, halved
- 1/4 cup crumbled feta cheese (optional)
- Fresh parsley for garnish

Instructions:

1. In a large bowl, whisk together the buckwheat flour, water, egg, olive oil, thyme, and oregano until smooth.
2. Heat a non-stick skillet over medium heat and lightly grease with a little olive oil.
3. Pour 1/4 cup of the batter into the skillet, tilting the pan to spread the batter evenly.
4. Cook for 2-3 minutes, until the edges start to lift and the crepe is set, then flip and cook for another 1-2 minutes.
5. Repeat with the remaining batter, greasing the skillet as needed.
6. In another pan, sauté the spinach until wilted and warm the cherry tomatoes slightly.
7. Fill each crepe with spinach, cherry tomatoes, and feta cheese, if using.
8. Garnish with fresh parsley and serve warm.

Nutrition Info per Serving (Serves 4):

- Calories: 200
- Protein: 6g
- Carbohydrates: 24g
- Fiber: 4g
- Sugars: 2g
- Fat: 10g
- Saturated Fat: 2g

Cooking Time:

- **Total: 20 minutes**

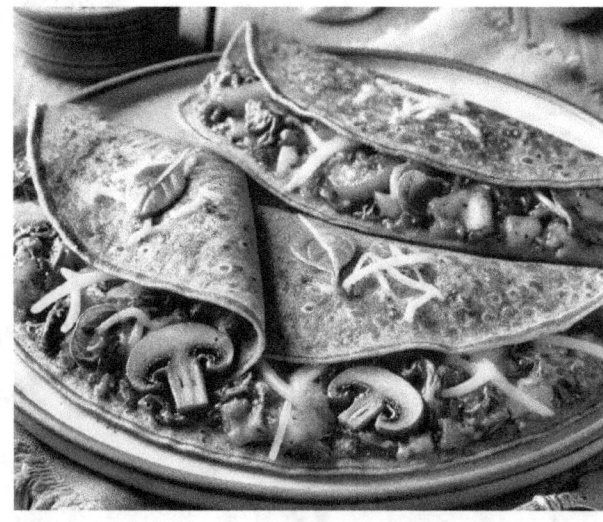

17. Pineapple and Spinach Green Juice

Ingredients:

- 2 cups fresh spinach
- 1 cup pineapple chunks (fresh or frozen)
- 1 cucumber, peeled and chopped
- 1 apple, cored and chopped
- 1 tablespoon lemon juice
- 1 cup water

Instructions:

1. In a blender, combine the spinach, pineapple chunks, cucumber, apple, lemon juice, and water.
2. Blend until smooth.
3. Pour through a fine-mesh strainer or cheesecloth into a pitcher, pressing down to extract as much juice as possible.
4. Serve immediately over ice or chilled.

Nutrition Info per Serving (Serves 2):

- Calories: 100
- Protein: 2g
- Carbohydrates: 25g
- Fiber: 3g
- Sugars: 15g
- Fat: 0.5g
- Saturated Fat: 0g

Cooking Time:

- **Total: 10 minutes**

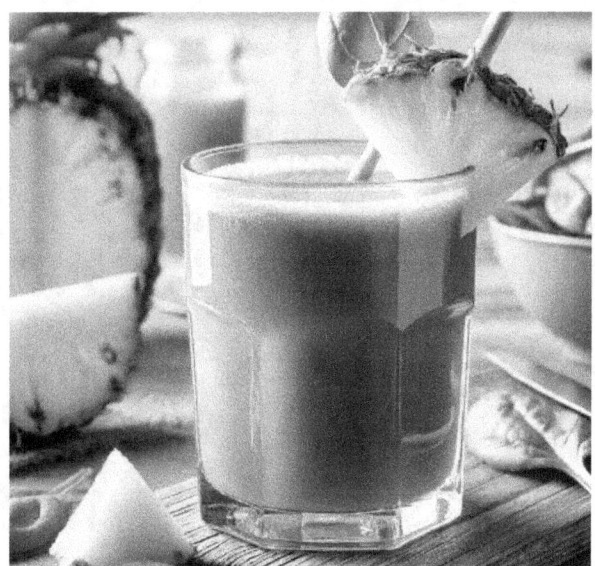

18. Herbed Chicken Patties

Ingredients:

- 1 pound ground chicken
- 1/4 cup finely chopped onion
- 2 cloves garlic, minced
- 1 tablespoon fresh parsley, chopped
- 1 tablespoon fresh dill, chopped
- 1 teaspoon dried oregano
- 1 egg, beaten
- 2 tablespoons almond flour
- 1 tablespoon olive oil

Instructions:

1. In a large bowl, combine the ground chicken, onion, garlic, parsley, dill, oregano, beaten egg, and almond flour. Mix well.
2. Form the mixture into small patties, about 2 inches in diameter.
3. Heat olive oil in a non-stick skillet over medium heat.
4. Cook the patties for about 4-5 minutes on each side, or until golden brown and cooked through.
5. Serve warm with a side salad or vegetables.

Nutrition Info per Serving (Serves 4):

- Calories: 220
- Protein: 20g
- Carbohydrates: 2g
- Fiber: 0.5g
- Sugars: 0g
- Fat: 15g
- Saturated Fat: 3g

Cooking Time:

- **Total: 20 minutes**

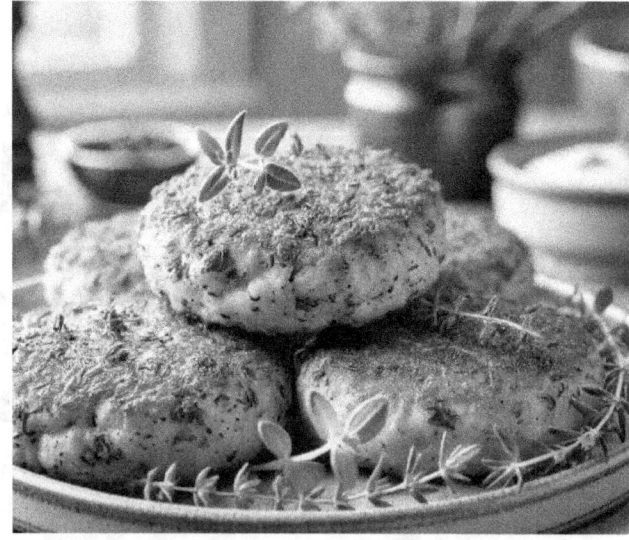

19. Green Tea with Lemon and Honey

Ingredients:

- 1 green tea bag
- 1 cup boiling water
- 1 tablespoon lemon juice
- 1 teaspoon honey

Instructions:

1. Place the green tea bag in a cup and pour boiling water over it.
2. Let the tea steep for 3-5 minutes, then remove the tea bag.
3. Stir in the lemon juice and honey until well combined.
4. Serve hot.

Nutrition Info per Serving (Serves 1):

- Calories: 20
- Protein: 0g
- Carbohydrates: 5g
- Fiber: 0g
- Sugars: 5g
- Fat: 0g
- Saturated Fat: 0g

Cooking Time:

- **Total: 5 minutes**

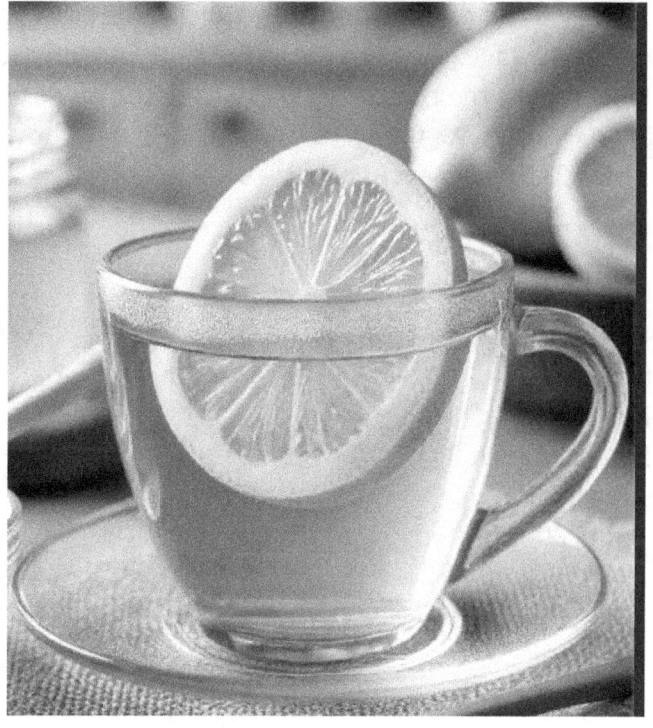

20. Flaxseed and Banana Pancakes

Ingredients:

- 1 cup almond flour
- 1/4 cup ground flaxseeds
- 1 teaspoon baking powder
- 1 teaspoon ground cinnamon
- 2 eggs
- 1 ripe banana, mashed
- 1/2 cup unsweetened almond milk
- 1 tablespoon coconut oil for cooking

Instructions:

1. In a large bowl, whisk together the almond flour, ground flaxseeds, baking powder, and ground cinnamon.
2. In another bowl, mix the eggs, mashed banana, and almond milk until well combined.
3. Pour the wet ingredients into the dry ingredients and stir until just combined.
4. Heat a small amount of coconut oil in a non-stick skillet over medium heat.
5. Pour 1/4 cup of batter onto the skillet for each pancake. Cook until bubbles form on the surface, then flip and cook until golden brown on the other side.
6. Repeat with the remaining batter, adding more coconut oil as needed.
7. Serve warm with fresh fruit or a drizzle of honey.

Nutrition Info per Serving (Serves 4):

- Calories: 230
- Protein: 8g
- Carbohydrates: 18g
- Fiber: 6g
- Sugars: 6g
- Fat: 15g
- Saturated Fat: 3g

Cooking Time:

- **Total: 20 minutes**

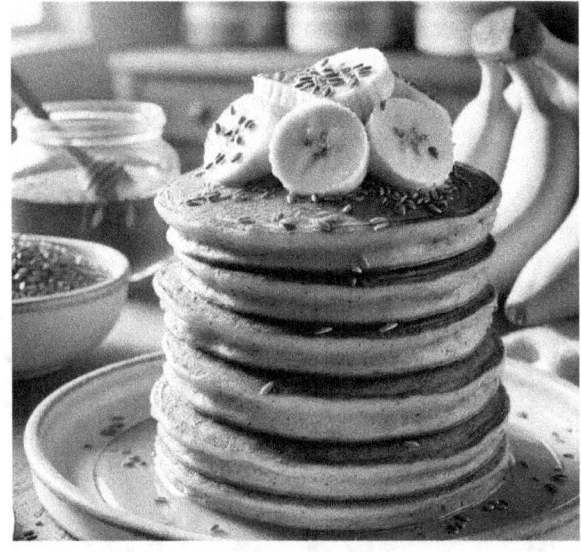

21. Kefir with Honey and Almonds

Ingredients:

- 1 cup plain kefir
- 1 tablespoon honey
- 2 tablespoons sliced almonds
- 1/4 teaspoon ground cinnamon

Instructions:

1. Pour the kefir into a bowl.
2. Drizzle with honey.
3. Sprinkle with sliced almonds and ground cinnamon.
4. Stir gently to combine and serve immediately.

Nutrition Info per Serving (Serves 1):

- Calories: 200
- Protein: 8g
- Carbohydrates: 24g
- Fiber: 2g
- Sugars: 18g
- Fat: 8g
- Saturated Fat: 1g

Cooking Time:

- **Total: 5 minutes**

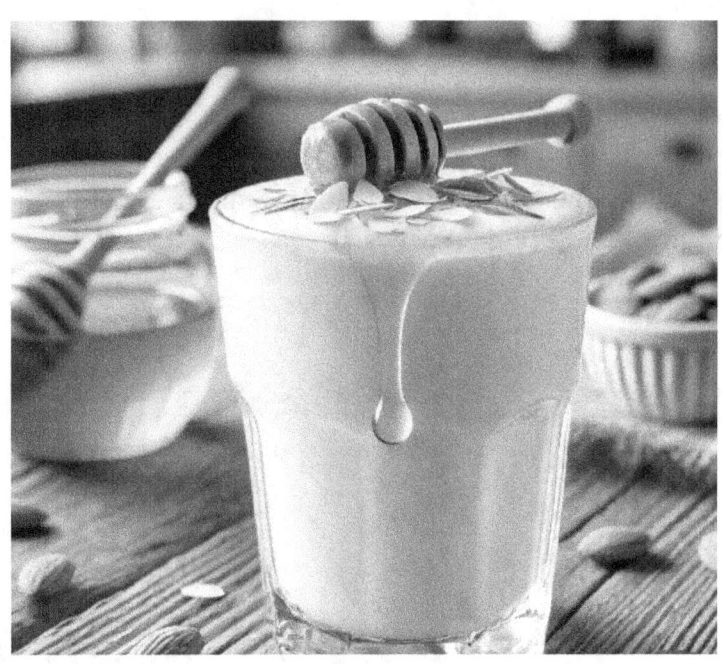

Poultry Recipes

1. Herb-Roasted Chicken Breast

Ingredients:

- 4 boneless, skinless chicken breasts
- 2 tablespoons olive oil
- 1 tablespoon fresh rosemary, chopped
- 1 tablespoon fresh thyme, chopped
- 1 tablespoon fresh parsley, chopped
- 2 cloves garlic, minced
- 1 lemon, sliced
- 1 teaspoon paprika

Instructions:

1. Preheat the oven to 375°F (190°C).
2. In a small bowl, mix together the olive oil, rosemary, thyme, parsley, garlic, and paprika.
3. Place the chicken breasts in a baking dish and rub the herb mixture over them.
4. Arrange the lemon slices on top of the chicken.
5. Bake for 25-30 minutes, or until the chicken is cooked through and no longer pink in the center.
6. Remove from the oven and let rest for 5 minutes before serving.

Nutrition Info per Serving (Serves 4):

- Calories: 250
- Protein: 26g
- Carbohydrates: 2g
- Fiber: 1g
- Sugars: 0g
- Fat: 15g
- Saturated Fat: 2g

Cooking Time:

- **Total: 35 minutes**

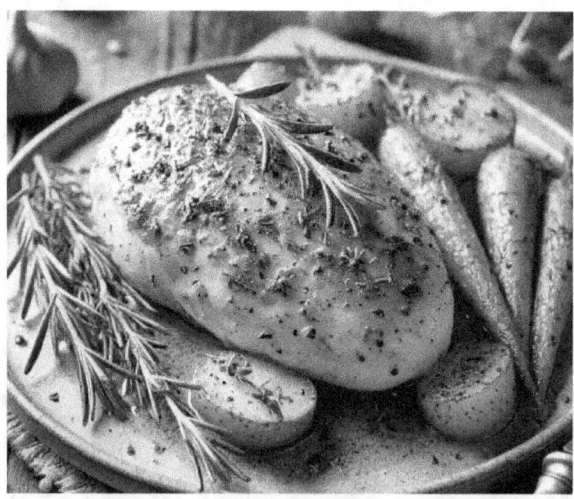

2. Chicken Soup with Vegetables

Ingredients:

- 1 tablespoon olive oil
- 1 medium onion, chopped
- 2 cloves garlic, minced
- 3 carrots, peeled and sliced
- 2 celery stalks, sliced
- 1 zucchini, diced
- 1 pound boneless, skinless chicken breasts, cut into bite-sized pieces
- 6 cups low-sodium chicken broth
- 1 teaspoon dried thyme
- 1 teaspoon dried oregano
- Fresh parsley for garnish

Instructions:

1. In a large pot, heat the olive oil over medium heat.
2. Add the onion and garlic, and cook for 3-4 minutes until softened.
3. Add the carrots, celery, zucchini, and chicken pieces. Cook for 5-7 minutes, stirring occasionally.
4. Pour in the chicken broth and add the thyme and oregano.
5. Bring to a boil, then reduce heat and simmer for 20-25 minutes, until the vegetables are tender and the chicken is cooked through.
6. Garnish with fresh parsley and serve warm.

Nutrition Info per Serving (Serves 6):

- Calories: 180
- Protein: 20g
- Carbohydrates: 10g
- Fiber: 2g
- Sugars: 4g
- Fat: 7g
- Saturated Fat: 1g

Cooking Time:

- **Total: 40 minutes**

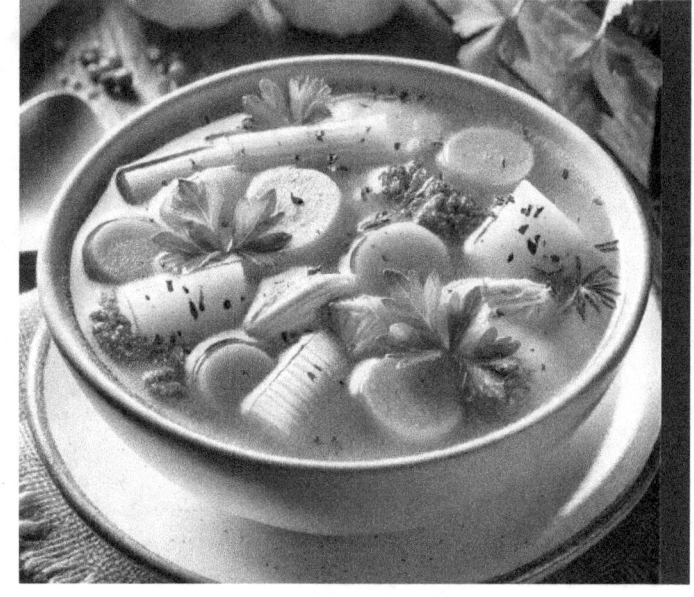

3. Lemon Garlic Turkey Cutlets

Ingredients:

- 1 pound turkey cutlets
- 2 tablespoons olive oil
- 3 cloves garlic, minced
- Juice of 1 lemon
- 1 teaspoon dried oregano
- 1 teaspoon paprika
- Fresh parsley for garnish

Instructions:

1. In a small bowl, mix together the olive oil, garlic, lemon juice, oregano, and paprika.
2. Rub the mixture over the turkey cutlets.
3. Heat a non-stick skillet over medium heat.
4. Cook the turkey cutlets for 3-4 minutes on each side, or until golden brown and cooked through.
5. Garnish with fresh parsley and serve immediately.

Nutrition Info per Serving (Serves 4):

- Calories: 210
- Protein: 28g
- Carbohydrates: 2g
- Fiber: 0g
- Sugars: 0g
- Fat: 10g
- Saturated Fat: 2g

Cooking Time:

- **Total: 15 minutes**

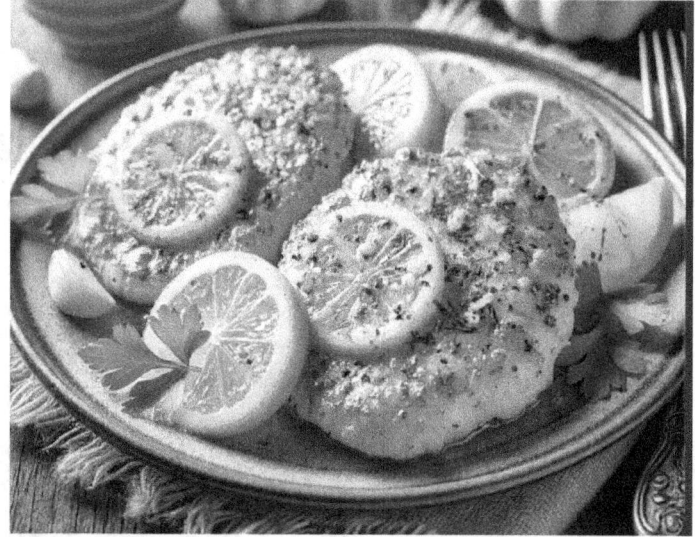

4. Baked Chicken with Brussels Sprouts

Ingredients:

- 4 boneless, skinless chicken thighs
- 1 pound Brussels sprouts, trimmed and halved
- 2 tablespoons olive oil
- 1 teaspoon dried thyme
- 1 teaspoon dried rosemary
- 1 teaspoon paprika
- 2 cloves garlic, minced
- 1 lemon, sliced

Instructions:

1. Preheat the oven to 400°F (200°C).
2. In a large bowl, mix the Brussels sprouts with 1 tablespoon olive oil, thyme, and rosemary.
3. Spread the Brussels sprouts in a single layer on a baking sheet.
4. In the same bowl, mix the chicken thighs with the remaining olive oil, paprika, and garlic.
5. Place the chicken thighs on top of the Brussels sprouts.
6. Arrange the lemon slices over the chicken.
7. Bake for 30-35 minutes, or until the chicken is cooked through and the Brussels sprouts are tender.
8. Serve warm.

Nutrition Info per Serving (Serves 4):

- Calories: 300
- Protein: 25g
- Carbohydrates: 10g
- Fiber: 4g
- Sugars: 2g
- Fat: 18g
- Saturated Fat: 4g

Cooking Time:

- **Total: 40 minutes**

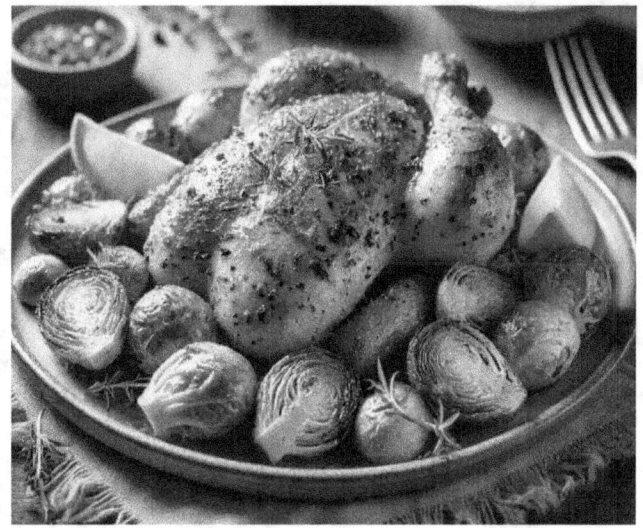

5. Chicken and Broccoli Stir-Fry

Ingredients:

- 1 pound boneless, skinless chicken breasts, cut into strips
- 2 tablespoons olive oil
- 3 cups broccoli florets
- 1 red bell pepper, sliced
- 1 yellow bell pepper, sliced
- 3 cloves garlic, minced
- 1 tablespoon fresh ginger, grated
- 1/4 cup low-sodium soy sauce
- 2 tablespoons honey
- 1 tablespoon sesame seeds (optional)

Instructions:

1. Heat 1 tablespoon of olive oil in a large skillet or wok over medium-high heat.
2. Add the chicken strips and cook for 5-7 minutes, until golden brown and cooked through. Remove from the skillet and set aside.
3. In the same skillet, heat the remaining olive oil.
4. Add the broccoli, red bell pepper, yellow bell pepper, garlic, and ginger. Cook for 5-7 minutes, stirring frequently, until the vegetables are tender-crisp.
5. In a small bowl, mix the soy sauce and honey.
6. Return the chicken to the skillet and pour the soy sauce mixture over the chicken and vegetables.
7. Cook for another 2-3 minutes, stirring to coat everything evenly.
8. Sprinkle with sesame seeds, if using, and serve immediately.

Nutrition Info per Serving (Serves 4):

- Calories: 260
- Protein: 28g
- Carbohydrates: 18g
- Fiber: 4g
- Sugars: 10g
- Fat: 9g
- Saturated Fat: 1.5g

Cooking Time:

- **Total: 20 minutes**

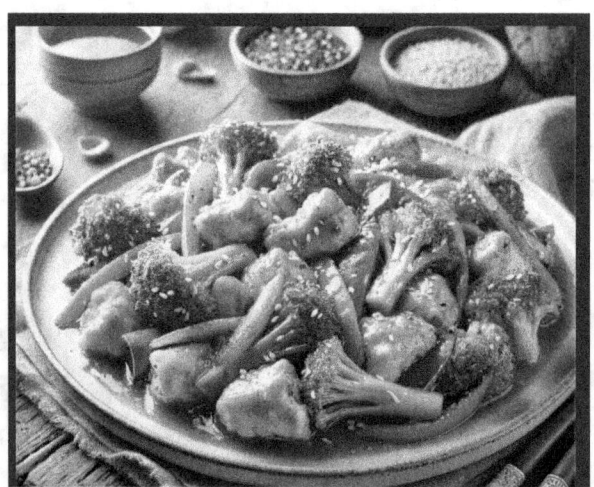

6. One-Pan Turmeric Chicken and Rice

Ingredients:

- 4 boneless, skinless chicken thighs
- 1 cup basmati rice, rinsed
- 2 cups low-sodium chicken broth
- 1 onion, chopped
- 2 cloves garlic, minced
- 1 teaspoon ground turmeric
- 1 teaspoon ground cumin
- 1 teaspoon paprika
- 1 tablespoon olive oil
- Fresh cilantro for garnish

Instructions:

1. Preheat the oven to 375°F (190°C).
2. In a large ovenproof skillet, heat the olive oil over medium heat.
3. Add the chopped onion and garlic, and cook for 3-4 minutes until softened.
4. Stir in the turmeric, cumin, and paprika, and cook for another minute.
5. Add the rice and stir to coat with the spices.
6. Pour in the chicken broth and bring to a boil.
7. Place the chicken thighs on top of the rice mixture.
8. Cover the skillet with a lid or aluminum foil and transfer to the oven.
9. Bake for 25-30 minutes, or until the chicken is cooked through and the rice is tender.
10. Garnish with fresh cilantro before serving.

Nutrition Info per Serving (Serves 4):

- Calories: 360
- Protein: 25g
- Carbohydrates: 40g
- Fiber: 2g
- Sugars: 2g
- Fat: 12g
- Saturated Fat: 2g

Cooking Time:

- **Total: 40 minutes**

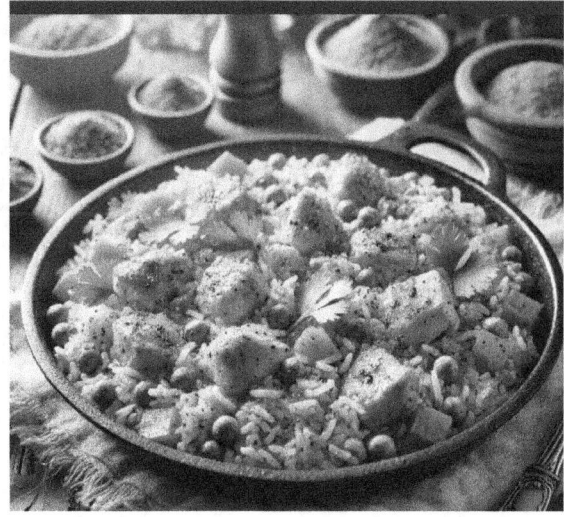

7. Turkey and Sweet Potato Skillet

Ingredients:

- 1 pound ground turkey
- 2 medium sweet potatoes, peeled and diced
- 1 bell pepper, chopped
- 1 onion, chopped
- 2 cloves garlic, minced
- 1 tablespoon olive oil
- 1 teaspoon ground cumin
- 1 teaspoon paprika
- Fresh parsley for garnish

Instructions:

1. Heat the olive oil in a large skillet over medium heat.
2. Add the onion and garlic, and cook for 3-4 minutes until softened.
3. Add the ground turkey and cook for 5-7 minutes, until browned and cooked through.
4. Stir in the diced sweet potatoes, bell pepper, cumin, and paprika.
5. Cover the skillet and cook for 10-12 minutes, stirring occasionally, until the sweet potatoes are tender.
6. Garnish with fresh parsley before serving.

Nutrition Info per Serving (Serves 4):

- Calories: 320
- Protein: 24g
- Carbohydrates: 30g
- Fiber: 5g
- Sugars: 7g
- Fat: 12g
- Saturated Fat: 2g

Cooking Time:

- **Total: 25 minutes**

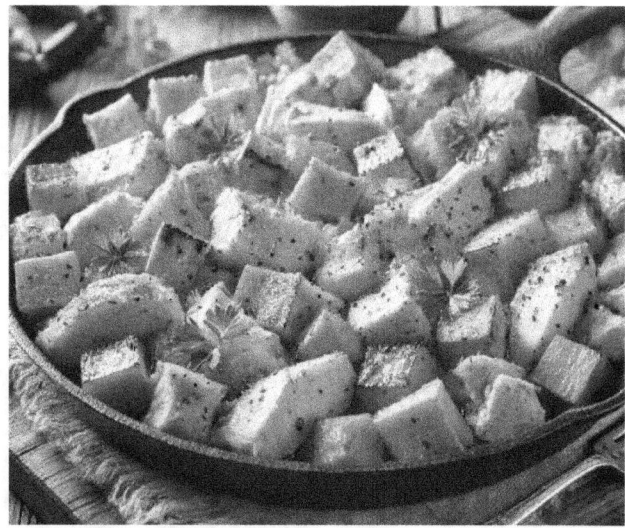

8. Rosemary Chicken Skewers

Ingredients:

- 1 pound boneless, skinless chicken breasts, cut into cubes
- 2 tablespoons olive oil
- 2 tablespoons fresh rosemary, chopped
- 2 cloves garlic, minced
- Juice of 1 lemon
- Wooden skewers, soaked in water

Instructions:

1. In a large bowl, mix together the olive oil, rosemary, garlic, and lemon juice.
2. Add the chicken cubes and toss to coat. Let marinate for at least 30 minutes.
3. Preheat the grill or a grill pan over medium-high heat.
4. Thread the marinated chicken onto the soaked wooden skewers.
5. Grill the skewers for 10-12 minutes, turning occasionally, until the chicken is cooked through.
6. Serve warm.

Nutrition Info per Serving (Serves 4):

- Calories: 200
- Protein: 25g
- Carbohydrates: 2g
- Fiber: 0.5g
- Sugars: 0g
- Fat: 10g
- Saturated Fat: 2g

Cooking Time:

- **Total: 45 minutes (including marinating time)**

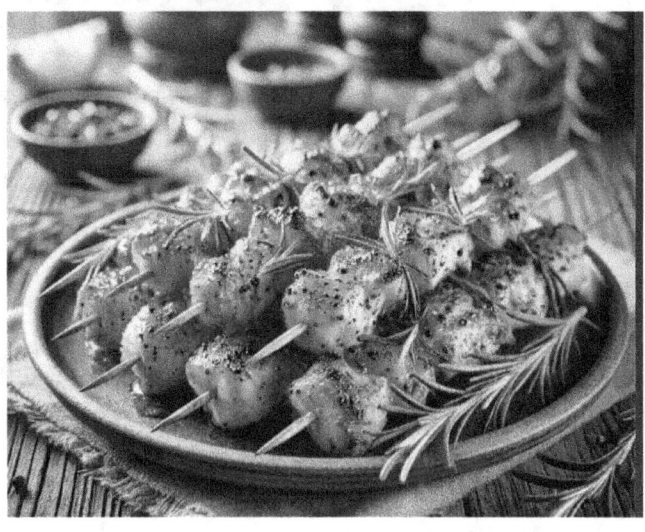

9. Slow Cooker Turkey Soup

Ingredients:

- 1 pound ground turkey
- 4 cups low-sodium chicken broth
- 2 carrots, peeled and sliced
- 2 celery stalks, sliced
- 1 onion, chopped
- 2 cloves garlic, minced
- 1 zucchini, diced
- 1 teaspoon dried thyme
- 1 teaspoon dried oregano
- Fresh parsley for garnish

Instructions:

1. In a skillet, cook the ground turkey over medium heat until browned.
2. Transfer the cooked turkey to a slow cooker.
3. Add the chicken broth, carrots, celery, onion, garlic, zucchini, thyme, and oregano.
4. Cover and cook on low for 6-8 hours, or on high for 3-4 hours, until the vegetables are tender.
5. Garnish with fresh parsley before serving.

Nutrition Info per Serving (Serves 6):

- Calories: 180
- Protein: 20g
- Carbohydrates: 12g
- Fiber: 3g
- Sugars: 5g
- Fat: 7g
- Saturated Fat: 1g

Cooking Time:
Total: 6-8 hours (slow cooker)

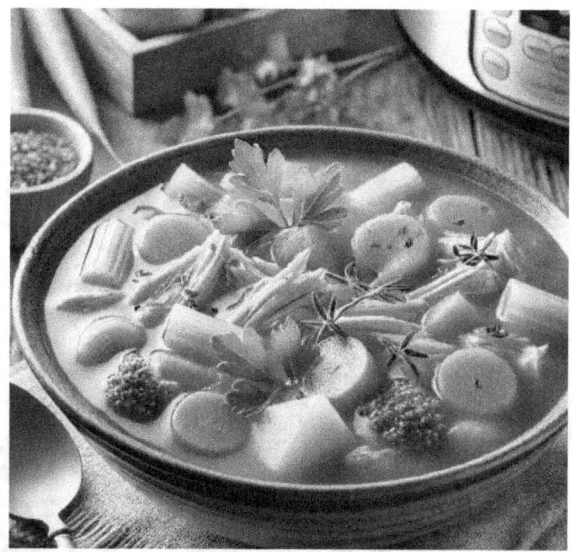

10. Chicken Apple Sausages

Ingredients:

- 1 pound ground chicken
- 1 apple, peeled and grated
- 1 small onion, finely chopped
- 2 cloves garlic, minced
- 1 tablespoon fresh sage, chopped
- 1 tablespoon fresh thyme, chopped
- 1 teaspoon ground nutmeg
- 1 tablespoon olive oil

Instructions:

1. In a large bowl, mix together the ground chicken, grated apple, onion, garlic, sage, thyme, and nutmeg.
2. Form the mixture into small patties or sausage links.
3. Heat the olive oil in a non-stick skillet over medium heat.
4. Cook the patties or sausages for 4-5 minutes on each side, or until golden brown and cooked through.
5. Serve warm.

Nutrition Info per Serving (Serves 4):

- Calories: 220
- Protein: 24g
- Carbohydrates: 6g
- Fiber: 1g
- Sugars: 4g
- Fat: 12g
- Saturated Fat: 2g

Cooking Time:

- **Total: 20 minutes**

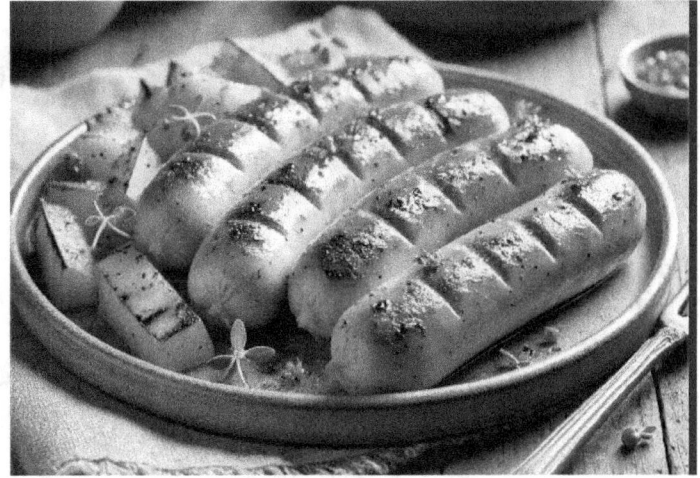

11. Turkey Meatloaf

Ingredients:

- 1 pound ground turkey
- 1 small onion, finely chopped
- 1 carrot, grated
- 2 cloves garlic, minced
- 1/2 cup rolled oats, finely ground
- 1 egg, beaten
- 1/4 cup unsweetened applesauce
- 1 tablespoon Dijon mustard
- 1 tablespoon Worcestershire sauce
- 1 teaspoon dried thyme
- 1 teaspoon dried oregano
- 1/4 cup tomato sauce

Instructions:

1. Preheat the oven to 375°F (190°C).
2. In a large bowl, combine the ground turkey, onion, carrot, garlic, ground oats, egg, applesauce, Dijon mustard, Worcestershire sauce, thyme, and oregano. Mix well.
3. Press the mixture into a loaf pan and top with tomato sauce.
4. Bake for 45-50 minutes, or until the internal temperature reaches 165°F (74°C).
5. Let rest for 5 minutes before slicing and serving.

Nutrition Info per Serving (Serves 4):

- Calories: 250
- Protein: 25g
- Carbohydrates: 15g
- Fiber: 2g
- Sugars: 6g
- Fat: 10g
- Saturated Fat: 2g

Cooking Time:

- **Total: 55 minutes**

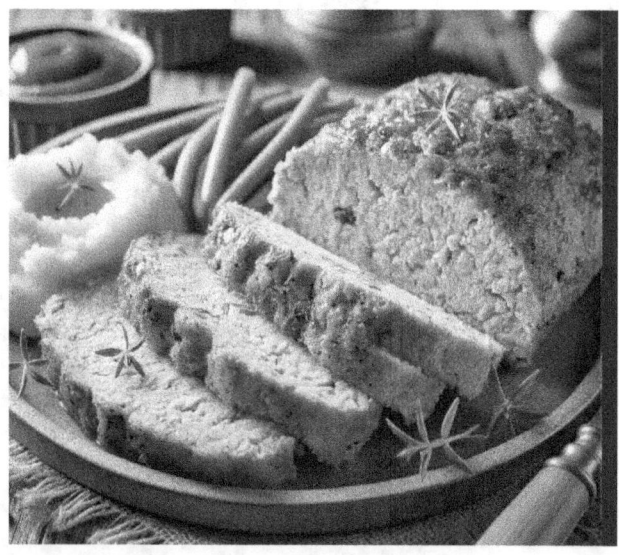

12. Roasted Turkey Breast with Herbs

Ingredients:

- 1 boneless turkey breast (about 2 pounds)
- 2 tablespoons olive oil
- 2 cloves garlic, minced
- 1 tablespoon fresh rosemary, chopped
- 1 tablespoon fresh thyme, chopped
- 1 tablespoon fresh sage, chopped
- 1 lemon, sliced

Instructions:

1. Preheat the oven to 375°F (190°C).
2. In a small bowl, mix together the olive oil, garlic, rosemary, thyme, and sage.
3. Rub the herb mixture all over the turkey breast.
4. Place the turkey breast in a roasting pan and arrange the lemon slices on top.
5. Roast for 45-55 minutes, or until the internal temperature reaches 165°F (74°C).
6. Let rest for 10 minutes before slicing and serving.

Nutrition Info per Serving (Serves 6):

- Calories: 210
- Protein: 32g
- Carbohydrates: 2g
- Fiber: 0.5g
- Sugars: 0.5g
- Fat: 8g
- Saturated Fat: 1.5g

Cooking Time:

- **Total: 65 minutes**

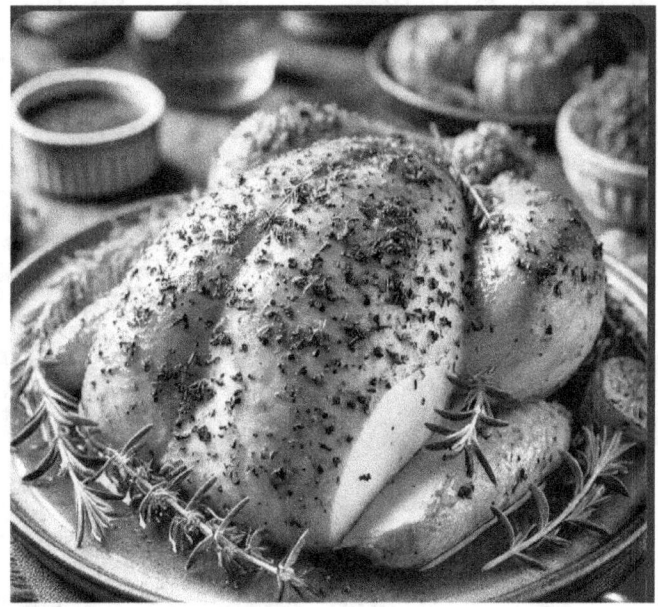

13. Asian-Inspired Chicken Salad

Ingredients:

- 2 boneless, skinless chicken breasts
- 4 cups mixed greens (spinach, arugula, kale)
- 1 cup shredded carrots
- 1 red bell pepper, thinly sliced
- 1/2 cup sliced almonds
- 2 green onions, chopped
- 1/4 cup sesame oil
- 2 tablespoons rice vinegar
- 1 tablespoon soy sauce (low sodium)
- 1 tablespoon honey
- 1 teaspoon fresh ginger, grated

Instructions:

1. Preheat a grill or grill pan over medium heat.
2. Grill the chicken breasts for 6-7 minutes on each side, or until fully cooked. Let cool and slice thinly.
3. In a large bowl, combine the mixed greens, shredded carrots, bell pepper, sliced almonds, and green onions.
4. In a small bowl, whisk together the sesame oil, rice vinegar, soy sauce, honey, and grated ginger.
5. Add the sliced chicken to the salad and toss with the dressing.
6. Serve immediately.

Nutrition Info per Serving (Serves 4):

- Calories: 300
- Protein: 25g
- Carbohydrates: 12g
- Fiber: 4g
- Sugars: 6g
- Fat: 18g
- Saturated Fat: 2.5g

Cooking Time:

- **Total: 20 minutes**

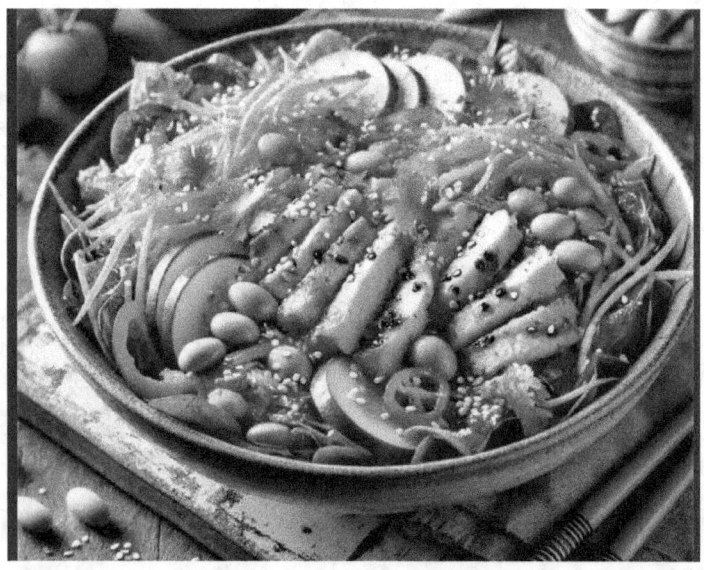

14. Balsamic Glazed Turkey Breast

Ingredients:

- 1 boneless turkey breast (about 2 pounds)
- 1/2 cup balsamic vinegar
- 1/4 cup honey
- 2 cloves garlic, minced
- 1 tablespoon olive oil
- 1 teaspoon dried thyme

Instructions:

1. Preheat the oven to 375°F (190°C).
2. In a small bowl, mix together the balsamic vinegar, honey, garlic, olive oil, and thyme.
3. Place the turkey breast in a roasting pan and brush with half of the balsamic mixture.
4. Roast for 45-55 minutes, basting with the remaining balsamic mixture halfway through, until the internal temperature reaches 165°F (74°C).
5. Let rest for 10 minutes before slicing and serving.

Nutrition Info per Serving (Serves 6):

- Calories: 220
- Protein: 32g
- Carbohydrates: 14g
- Fiber: 0.5g
- Sugars: 12g
- Fat: 6g
- Saturated Fat: 1g

Cooking Time:

- **Total: 65 minutes**

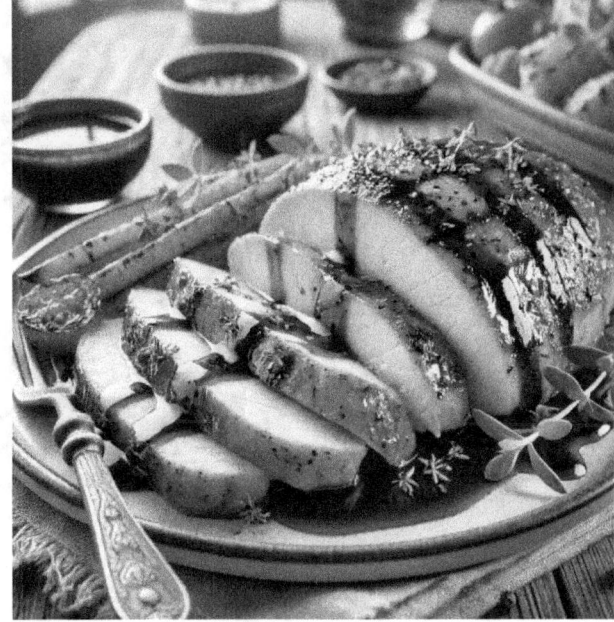

15. Chicken Vegetable Kabobs

Ingredients:

- 1 pound boneless, skinless chicken breasts, cut into cubes
- 1 red bell pepper, cut into chunks
- 1 yellow bell pepper, cut into chunks
- 1 zucchini, sliced
- 1 red onion, cut into chunks
- 2 tablespoons olive oil
- 2 cloves garlic, minced
- 1 teaspoon dried oregano
- Wooden skewers, soaked in water

Instructions:

1. In a large bowl, mix together the olive oil, garlic, and oregano.
2. Add the chicken cubes and vegetables, and toss to coat.
3. Preheat the grill or a grill pan over medium-high heat.
4. Thread the chicken and vegetables onto the soaked wooden skewers.
5. Grill the kabobs for 10-12 minutes, turning occasionally, until the chicken is cooked through and the vegetables are tender.
6. Serve warm.

Nutrition Info per Serving (Serves 4):

- Calories: 210
- Protein: 26g
- Carbohydrates: 8g
- Fiber: 2g
- Sugars: 4g
- Fat: 9g
- Saturated Fat: 1.5g

Cooking Time:

- **Total: 25 minutes**

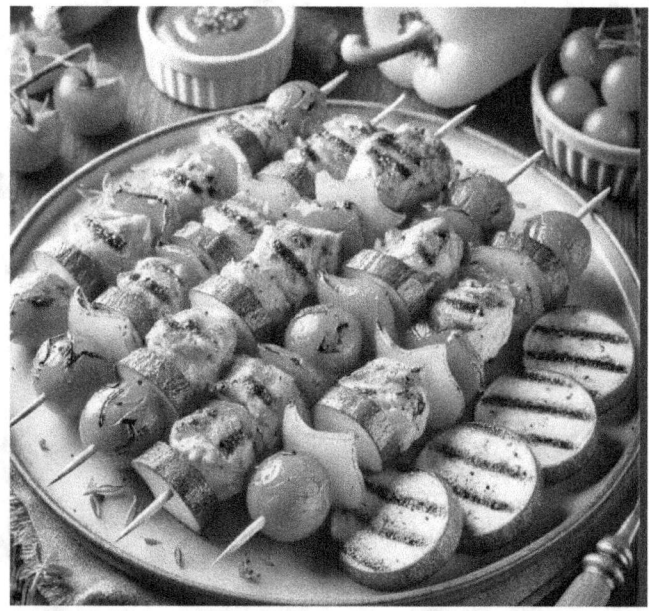

16. Turkey and Spinach Stuffed Mushrooms

Ingredients:

- 12 large white mushrooms, stems removed and chopped
- 1/2 pound ground turkey
- 1 cup fresh spinach, chopped
- 1/2 cup onion, finely chopped
- 2 cloves garlic, minced
- 1/4 cup almond flour
- 1 tablespoon olive oil
- 1 teaspoon dried thyme
- Fresh parsley for garnish

Instructions:

1. Preheat the oven to 375°F (190°C).
2. In a skillet, heat the olive oil over medium heat.
3. Add the chopped mushroom stems, onion, and garlic, and cook for 3-4 minutes until softened.
4. Add the ground turkey, chopped spinach, and thyme. Cook for another 5-7 minutes, until the turkey is cooked through.
5. Stir in the almond flour and mix well.
6. Fill each mushroom cap with the turkey mixture and place on a baking sheet.
7. Bake for 15-20 minutes, until the mushrooms are tender.
8. Garnish with fresh parsley and serve warm.

Nutrition Info per Serving (Serves 4):

- Calories: 170
- Protein: 20g
- Carbohydrates: 5g
- Fiber: 2g
- Sugars: 2g
- Fat: 8g
- Saturated Fat: 1.5g

Cooking Time:

- **Total: 30 minutes**

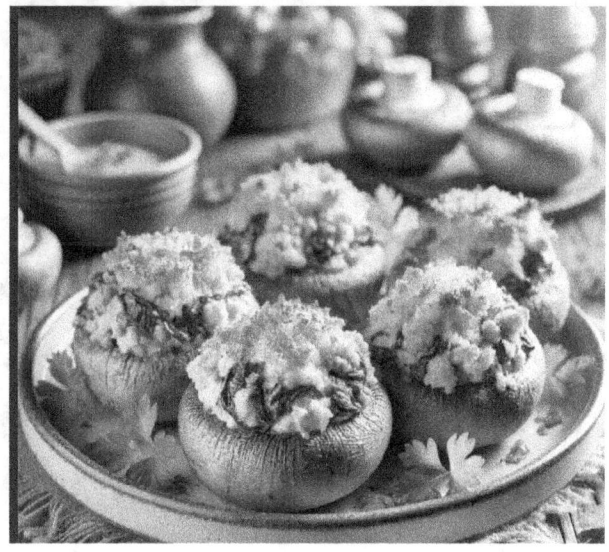

17. Grilled Chicken with Herb Salad

Ingredients:

- 4 boneless, skinless chicken breasts
- 2 tablespoons olive oil
- 2 cloves garlic, minced
- 1 teaspoon dried oregano
- 1 teaspoon dried thyme
- 4 cups mixed greens (arugula, spinach, kale)
- 1/2 cup fresh parsley, chopped
- 1/4 cup fresh mint, chopped
- 1/4 cup fresh basil, chopped
- 1/4 cup lemon juice
- 2 tablespoons olive oil

Instructions:

1. Preheat the grill to medium-high heat.
2. In a small bowl, mix 2 tablespoons olive oil, garlic, oregano, and thyme.
3. Brush the chicken breasts with the olive oil mixture.
4. Grill the chicken breasts for 6-7 minutes on each side, or until fully cooked.
5. In a large bowl, combine the mixed greens, parsley, mint, and basil.
6. In a small bowl, whisk together the lemon juice and 2 tablespoons olive oil. Pour over the salad and toss to coat.
7. Serve the grilled chicken with the herb salad.

Nutrition Info per Serving (Serves 4):

- Calories: 320
- Protein: 30g
- Carbohydrates: 6g
- Fiber: 3g
- Sugars: 1g
- Fat: 20g
- Saturated Fat: 3g

Cooking Time:

- **Total: 20 minutes**

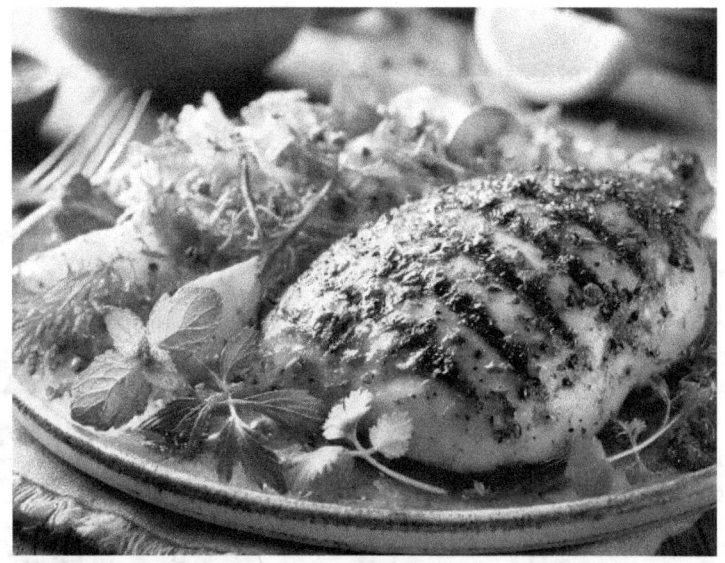

18. Poached Chicken with Avocado Salsa

Ingredients:

- 4 boneless, skinless chicken breasts
- 4 cups low-sodium chicken broth
- 1 avocado, diced
- 1 small red onion, finely chopped
- 1 jalapeno, seeded and minced
- 1/4 cup fresh cilantro, chopped
- 1 lime, juiced
- 1 tablespoon olive oil

Instructions:

1. In a large pot, bring the chicken broth to a simmer.
2. Add the chicken breasts and poach for 10-15 minutes, until fully cooked.
3. In a medium bowl, combine the avocado, red onion, jalapeno, cilantro, lime juice, and olive oil. Mix gently.
4. Remove the chicken breasts from the broth and let cool slightly.
5. Slice the chicken breasts and top with the avocado salsa.
6. Serve immediately.

Nutrition Info per Serving (Serves 4):

- Calories: 280
- Protein: 28g
- Carbohydrates: 10g
- Fiber: 5g
- Sugars: 2g
- Fat: 16g
- Saturated Fat: 2.5g

Cooking Time:

- **Total: 20 minutes**

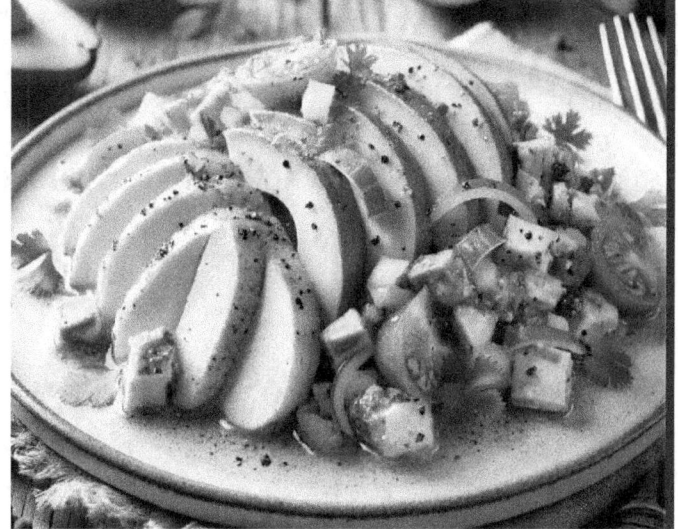

19. Turkey and Kale Soup

Ingredients:

- 1 tablespoon olive oil
- 1 pound ground turkey
- 1 onion, chopped
- 2 cloves garlic, minced
- 4 cups low-sodium chicken broth
- 2 carrots, peeled and sliced
- 2 celery stalks, sliced
- 2 cups chopped kale
- 1 teaspoon dried thyme
- 1 teaspoon dried oregano

Instructions:

1. In a large pot, heat the olive oil over medium heat.
2. Add the onion and garlic, and cook for 3-4 minutes until softened.
3. Add the ground turkey and cook until browned.
4. Stir in the chicken broth, carrots, celery, thyme, and oregano. Bring to a boil.
5. Reduce heat and simmer for 20 minutes, until the vegetables are tender.
6. Stir in the chopped kale and cook for an additional 5 minutes.
7. Serve warm.

Nutrition Info per Serving (Serves 6):

- Calories: 200
- Protein: 22g
- Carbohydrates: 10g
- Fiber: 3g
- Sugars: 4g
- Fat: 9g
- Saturated Fat: 2g

Cooking Time:

- **Total: 35 minutes**

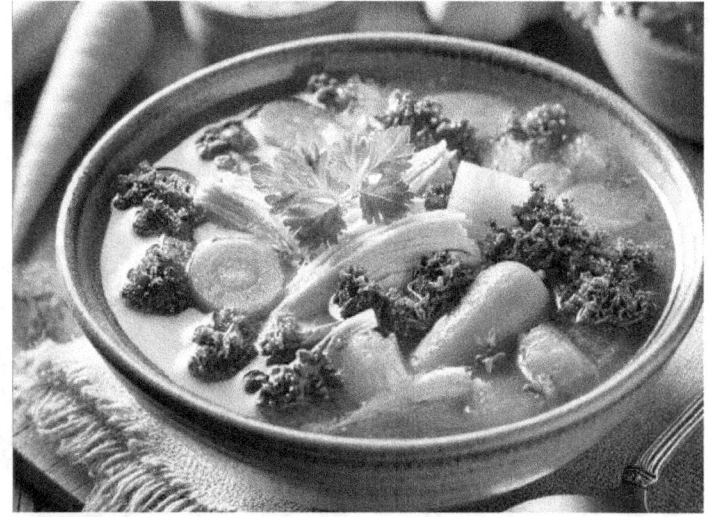

20. Turkey Spinach Mini Meatballs

Ingredients:

- 1 pound ground turkey
- 1 cup fresh spinach, finely chopped
- 1 small onion, finely chopped
- 2 cloves garlic, minced
- 1 egg, beaten
- 1/4 cup almond flour
- 1 teaspoon dried basil
- 1 teaspoon dried oregano
- 1 tablespoon olive oil

Instructions:

1. Preheat the oven to 375°F (190°C) and line a baking sheet with parchment paper.
2. In a large bowl, combine the ground turkey, spinach, onion, garlic, egg, almond flour, basil, and oregano. Mix well.
3. Form the mixture into small meatballs and place them on the prepared baking sheet.
4. Bake for 20-25 minutes, or until the meatballs are cooked through.
5. Heat the olive oil in a skillet over medium heat and brown the meatballs for 2-3 minutes for added flavor.
6. Serve warm.

Nutrition Info per Serving (Serves 4):

- Calories: 240
- Protein: 26g
- Carbohydrates: 6g
- Fiber: 2g
- Sugars: 1g
- Fat: 13g
- Saturated Fat: 2g

Cooking Time:

- **Total: 30 minutes**

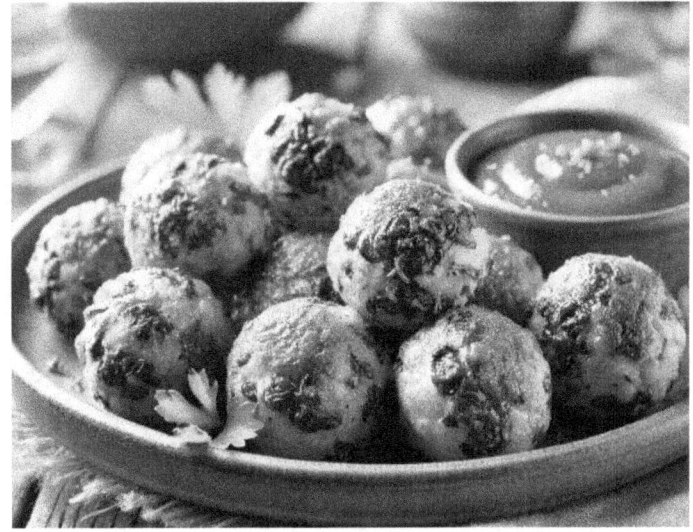

21. Spiced Chicken with Cauliflower

Ingredients:

- 4 boneless, skinless chicken thighs
- 1 head of cauliflower, cut into florets
- 2 tablespoons olive oil
- 1 teaspoon ground cumin
- 1 teaspoon ground coriander
- 1 teaspoon paprika
- 1/2 teaspoon ground turmeric
- Fresh cilantro for garnish

Instructions:

1. Preheat the oven to 400°F (200°C).
2. In a small bowl, mix together the olive oil, cumin, coriander, paprika, and turmeric.
3. Rub the spice mixture all over the chicken thighs.
4. Arrange the cauliflower florets on a baking sheet and drizzle with a little olive oil.
5. Place the chicken thighs on top of the cauliflower.
6. Roast for 25-30 minutes, or until the chicken is cooked through and the cauliflower is tender.
7. Garnish with fresh cilantro before serving.

Nutrition Info per Serving (Serves 4):

- Calories: 280
- Protein: 22g
- Carbohydrates: 10g
- Fiber: 4g
- Sugars: 3g
- Fat: 18g
- Saturated Fat: 3.5g

Cooking Time:

- **Total: 35 minutes**

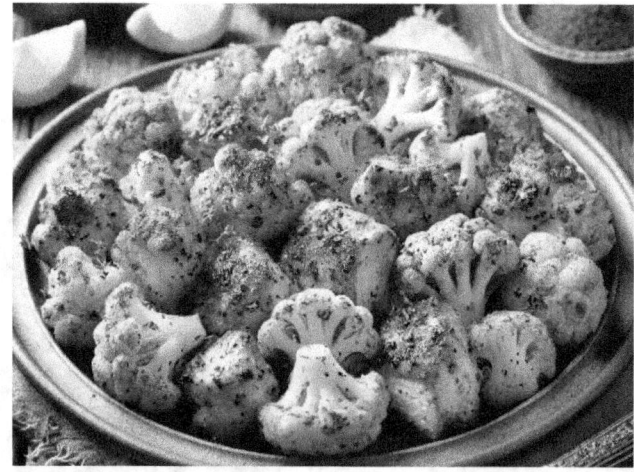

Meat Recipes

1. Beef Stir Fry with Broccoli

Ingredients:

- 1 pound beef sirloin, thinly sliced
- 3 cups broccoli florets
- 2 tablespoons olive oil
- 3 cloves garlic, minced
- 1 tablespoon fresh ginger, grated
- 1/4 cup low-sodium soy sauce
- 1 tablespoon honey
- 1 tablespoon sesame oil
- 1 tablespoon cornstarch mixed with 2 tablespoons water
- 1 tablespoon sesame seeds (optional)

Instructions:

1. Heat 1 tablespoon of olive oil in a large skillet or wok over medium-high heat.
2. Add the beef slices and stir-fry for 3-4 minutes until browned. Remove from the skillet and set aside.
3. In the same skillet, add the remaining olive oil, garlic, and ginger. Stir-fry for 1-2 minutes until fragrant.
4. Add the broccoli florets and stir-fry for 4-5 minutes until tender-crisp.
5. Return the beef to the skillet.
6. In a small bowl, mix the soy sauce, honey, sesame oil, and cornstarch mixture. Pour over the beef and broccoli.
7. Stir-fry for another 2-3 minutes until the sauce thickens and everything is well coated.
8. Garnish with sesame seeds, if using, and serve immediately.

Nutrition Info per Serving (Serves 4):

- Calories: 300
- Protein: 28g
- Carbohydrates: 12g
- Fiber: 3g
- Sugars: 5g
- Fat: 16g
- Saturated Fat: 4g

Cooking Time:

- **Total: 20 minutes**

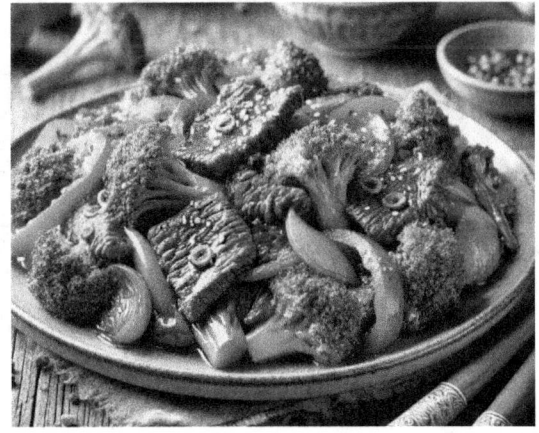

2. Lamb and Spinach Curry

Ingredients:

- 1 pound lamb, cut into cubes
- 2 tablespoons olive oil
- 1 onion, chopped
- 3 cloves garlic, minced
- 1 tablespoon fresh ginger, grated
- 2 tablespoons curry powder
- 1 teaspoon ground cumin
- 1 teaspoon ground coriander
- 1 can (14 oz) coconut milk
- 2 cups fresh spinach, chopped
- Fresh cilantro for garnish

Instructions:

1. Heat the olive oil in a large pot over medium heat.
2. Add the onion, garlic, and ginger, and cook for 3-4 minutes until softened.
3. Add the lamb cubes and brown on all sides for 5-6 minutes.
4. Stir in the curry powder, cumin, and coriander, and cook for another 1-2 minutes.
5. Pour in the coconut milk and bring to a simmer.
6. Reduce heat and simmer for 25-30 minutes, until the lamb is tender.
7. Stir in the chopped spinach and cook for an additional 5 minutes.
8. Garnish with fresh cilantro and serve warm.

Nutrition Info per Serving (Serves 4):

- Calories: 400
- Protein: 25g
- Carbohydrates: 10g
- Fiber: 3g
- Sugars: 2g
- Fat: 30g
- Saturated Fat: 15g

Cooking Time:

- **Total: 45 minutes**

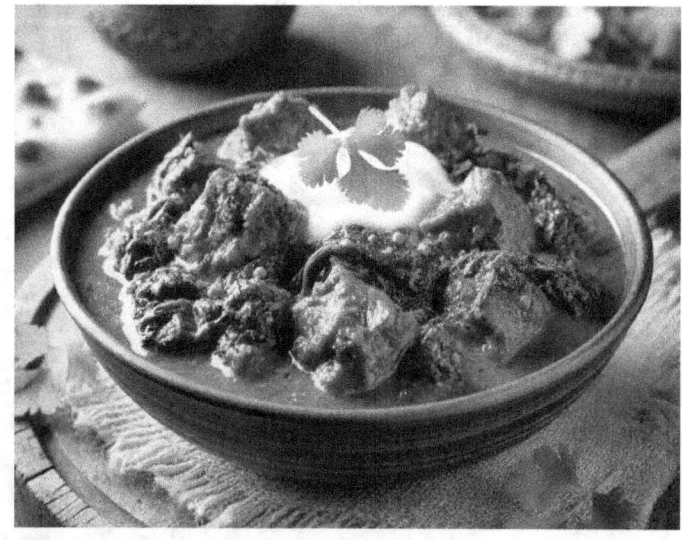

3. Grilled Sirloin Steak with Asparagus

Ingredients:

- 4 sirloin steaks (6 oz each)
- 2 tablespoons olive oil
- 2 cloves garlic, minced
- 1 teaspoon dried rosemary
- 1 pound asparagus, trimmed
- 1 lemon, sliced

Instructions:

1. Preheat the grill to medium-high heat.
2. In a small bowl, mix 1 tablespoon of olive oil, garlic, and rosemary.
3. Brush the mixture over the steaks.
4. Grill the steaks for 4-5 minutes on each side, or until desired doneness.
5. While the steaks are grilling, toss the asparagus with the remaining olive oil.
6. Grill the asparagus for 3-4 minutes, turning occasionally, until tender.
7. Serve the steaks with the grilled asparagus and lemon slices.

Nutrition Info per Serving (Serves 4):

- Calories: 350
- Protein: 40g
- Carbohydrates: 6g
- Fiber: 3g
- Sugars: 2g
- Fat: 18g
- Saturated Fat: 5g

Cooking Time:

- **Total: 20 minutes**

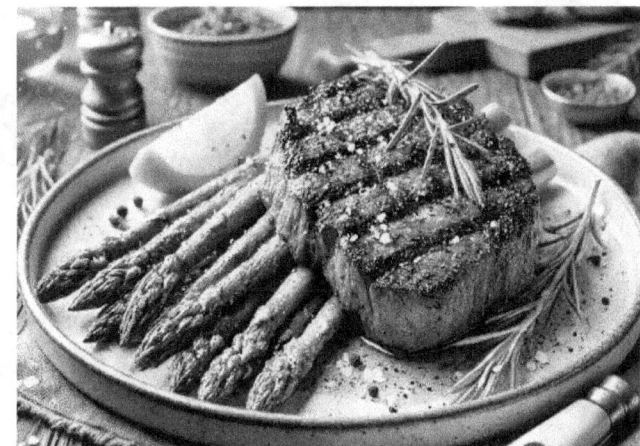

4. Spiced Lamb Kebabs

Ingredients:

- 1 pound ground lamb
- 1 small onion, finely chopped
- 2 cloves garlic, minced
- 1 tablespoon fresh parsley, chopped
- 1 tablespoon fresh mint, chopped
- 1 teaspoon ground cumin
- 1 teaspoon ground coriander
- 1 teaspoon paprika
- Wooden skewers, soaked in water

Instructions:

1. In a large bowl, mix together the ground lamb, onion, garlic, parsley, mint, cumin, coriander, and paprika.
2. Form the mixture into small sausage-shaped kebabs around the soaked wooden skewers.
3. Preheat the grill or grill pan over medium-high heat.
4. Grill the kebabs for 8-10 minutes, turning occasionally, until cooked through.
5. Serve warm.

Nutrition Info per Serving (Serves 4):

- Calories: 280
- Protein: 20g
- Carbohydrates: 5g
- Fiber: 1g
- Sugars: 1g
- Fat: 20g
- Saturated Fat: 8g

Cooking Time:

- **Total: 20 minutes**

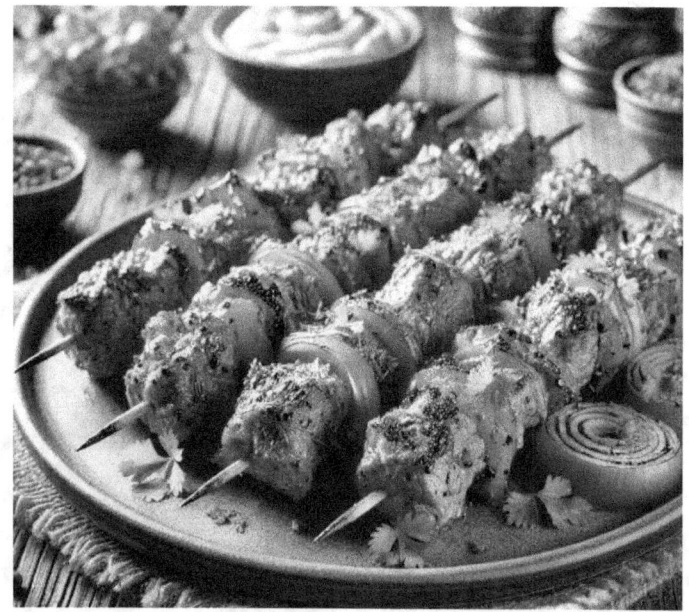

5. Pork Chops with Pear Sauce

Ingredients:

- 4 boneless pork chops
- 2 tablespoons olive oil
- 2 pears, peeled and sliced
- 1 small onion, finely chopped
- 2 cloves garlic, minced
- 1/2 cup low-sodium chicken broth
- 1 tablespoon honey
- 1 teaspoon dried thyme

Instructions:

1. Heat 1 tablespoon of olive oil in a large skillet over medium-high heat.
2. Add the pork chops and cook for 4-5 minutes on each side, until browned and cooked through. Remove from the skillet and set aside.
3. In the same skillet, add the remaining olive oil, pears, onion, and garlic. Cook for 3-4 minutes, until the onion is softened.
4. Stir in the chicken broth, honey, and thyme. Cook for another 5 minutes, until the sauce is slightly thickened.
5. Return the pork chops to the skillet and spoon the pear sauce over them.
6. Serve warm.

Nutrition Info per Serving (Serves 4):

- Calories: 350
- Protein: 28g
- Carbohydrates: 18g
- Fiber: 3g
- Sugars: 12g
- Fat: 18g
- Saturated Fat: 4g

Cooking Time:

- **Total: 25 minutes**

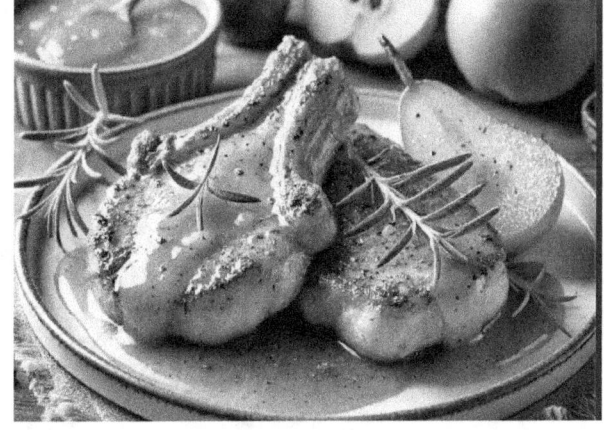

6. Beef and Vegetable Soup

Ingredients:

- 1 pound beef stew meat, cubed
- 2 tablespoons olive oil
- 1 onion, chopped
- 3 cloves garlic, minced
- 3 carrots, peeled and sliced
- 2 celery stalks, sliced
- 2 potatoes, diced
- 1 zucchini, diced
- 1 can (14.5 oz) diced tomatoes, no salt added
- 4 cups low-sodium beef broth
- 1 teaspoon dried thyme
- 1 teaspoon dried oregano
- Fresh parsley for garnish

Instructions:

1. In a large pot, heat olive oil over medium heat. Add the beef and brown on all sides, about 5-7 minutes.
2. Add the onion and garlic, and cook for 3-4 minutes until softened.
3. Stir in the carrots, celery, potatoes, zucchini, diced tomatoes, beef broth, thyme, and oregano.
4. Bring to a boil, then reduce heat and simmer for 45-50 minutes, until the vegetables are tender and the beef is cooked through.
5. Garnish with fresh parsley before serving.

Nutrition Info per Serving (Serves 6):

- Calories: 280
- Protein: 25g
- Carbohydrates: 20g
- Fiber: 4g
- Sugars: 5g
- Fat: 12g
- Saturated Fat: 3g

Cooking Time:

- **Total: 1 hour**

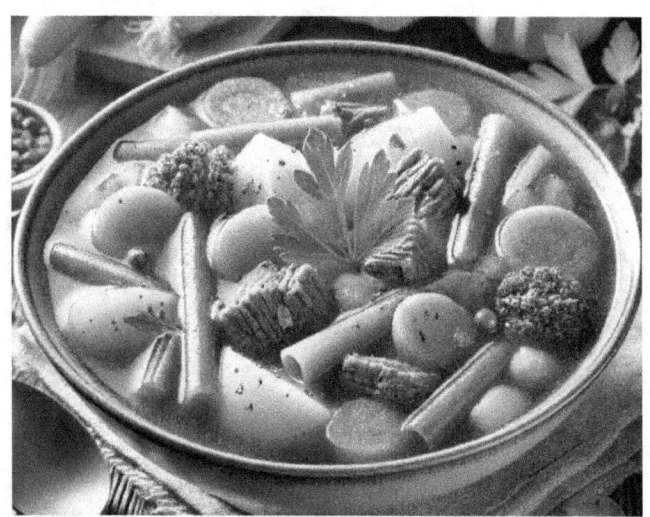

7. Lamb Stew with Turnips and Carrots

Ingredients:

- 1 pound lamb shoulder, cubed
- 2 tablespoons olive oil
- 1 onion, chopped
- 3 cloves garlic, minced
- 3 turnips, peeled and diced
- 3 carrots, peeled and sliced
- 4 cups low-sodium chicken broth
- 1 teaspoon dried rosemary
- 1 teaspoon dried thyme
- Fresh parsley for garnish

Instructions:

1. In a large pot, heat olive oil over medium heat. Add the lamb and brown on all sides, about 5-7 minutes.
2. Add the onion and garlic, and cook for 3-4 minutes until softened.
3. Stir in the turnips, carrots, chicken broth, rosemary, and thyme.
4. Bring to a boil, then reduce heat and simmer for 1 hour, until the lamb and vegetables are tender.
5. Garnish with fresh parsley before serving.

Nutrition Info per Serving (Serves 4):

- Calories: 350
- Protein: 28g
- Carbohydrates: 15g
- Fiber: 4g
- Sugars: 6g
- Fat: 20g
- Saturated Fat: 6g

Cooking Time:

- **Total: 1 hour 15 minutes**

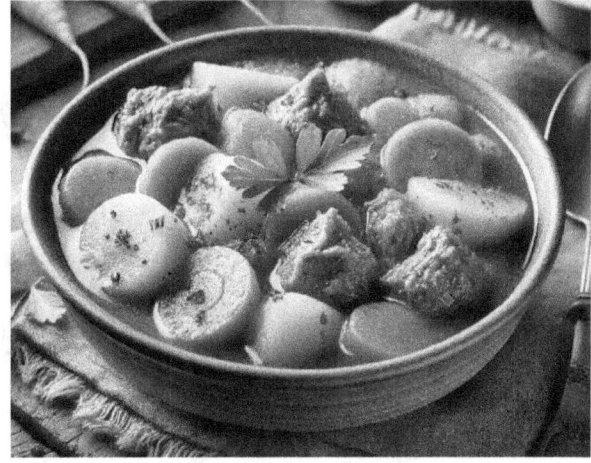

8. Grilled Lamb Chops with Mint Pesto

Ingredients:

- 8 lamb chops
- 2 tablespoons olive oil
- 2 cloves garlic, minced
- 1 cup fresh mint leaves
- 1/4 cup fresh parsley leaves
- 1/4 cup pine nuts
- 1/2 cup olive oil
- 2 tablespoons lemon juice

Instructions:

1. Preheat the grill to medium-high heat.
2. In a small bowl, mix 2 tablespoons of olive oil and garlic. Brush over the lamb chops.
3. Grill the lamb chops for 4-5 minutes on each side, or until desired doneness.
4. In a food processor, combine the mint leaves, parsley leaves, pine nuts, 1/2 cup olive oil, and lemon juice. Blend until smooth.
5. Serve the lamb chops with the mint pesto.

Nutrition Info per Serving (Serves 4):

- Calories: 450
- Protein: 25g
- Carbohydrates: 4g
- Fiber: 1g
- Sugars: 1g
- Fat: 38g
- Saturated Fat: 10g

Cooking Time:

- **Total: 20 minutes**

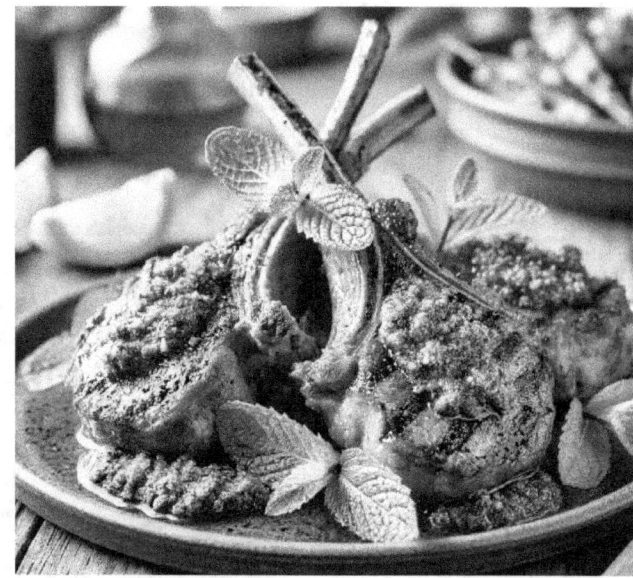

9. Beef Kabobs with Bell Peppers

Ingredients:

- 1 pound beef sirloin, cubed
- 2 tablespoons olive oil
- 1 teaspoon dried oregano
- 1 teaspoon paprika
- 1 red bell pepper, cut into chunks
- 1 yellow bell pepper, cut into chunks
- 1 green bell pepper, cut into chunks
- Wooden skewers, soaked in water

Instructions:

1. Preheat the grill to medium-high heat.
2. In a large bowl, mix the olive oil, oregano, and paprika. Add the beef and toss to coat.
3. Thread the beef and bell pepper chunks onto the soaked wooden skewers.
4. Grill the kabobs for 10-12 minutes, turning occasionally, until the beef is cooked through and the vegetables are tender.
5. Serve warm.

Nutrition Info per Serving (Serves 4):

- Calories: 300
- Protein: 26g
- Carbohydrates: 6g
- Fiber: 2g
- Sugars: 4g
- Fat: 18g
- Saturated Fat: 4g

Cooking Time:

- **Total: 20 minutes**

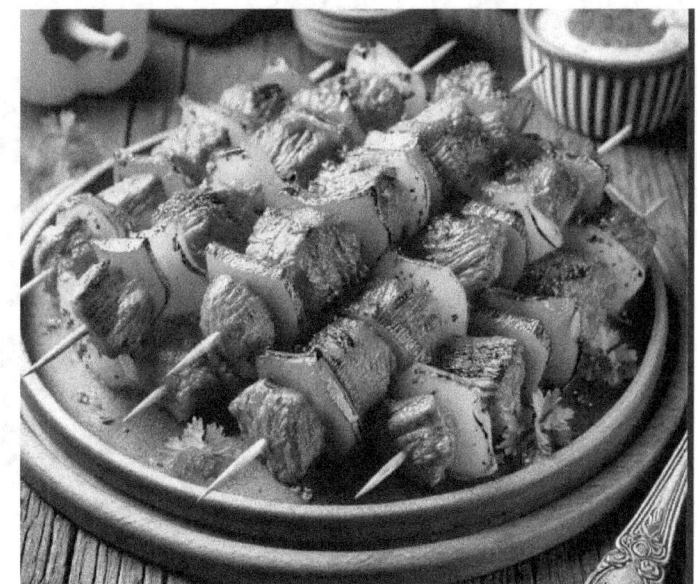

10. Lamb Soup with Barley and Mushrooms

Ingredients:

- 1 pound lamb shoulder, cubed
- 2 tablespoons olive oil
- 1 onion, chopped
- 3 cloves garlic, minced
- 1 cup pearl barley
- 8 cups low-sodium chicken broth
- 2 cups mushrooms, sliced
- 2 carrots, peeled and sliced
- 2 celery stalks, sliced
- 1 teaspoon dried thyme
- Fresh parsley for garnish

Instructions:

1. In a large pot, heat olive oil over medium heat. Add the lamb and brown on all sides, about 5-7 minutes.
2. Add the onion and garlic, and cook for 3-4 minutes until softened.
3. Stir in the pearl barley, chicken broth, mushrooms, carrots, celery, and thyme.
4. Bring to a boil, then reduce heat and simmer for 1 hour, until the lamb is tender and the barley is cooked.
5. Garnish with fresh parsley before serving.

Nutrition Info per Serving (Serves 6):

- Calories: 350
- Protein: 25g
- Carbohydrates: 35g
- Fiber: 8g
- Sugars: 6g
- Fat: 12g
- Saturated Fat: 3g

Cooking Time:

- **Total: 1 hour 15 minutes**

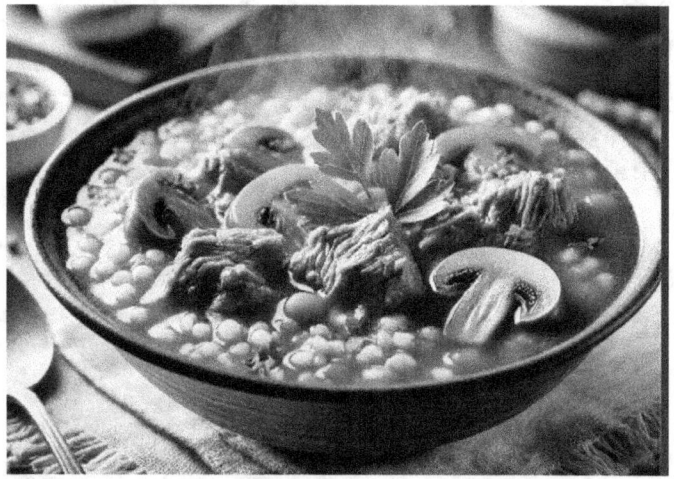

11. Pork Stir Fry with Snow Peas

Ingredients:

- 1 pound pork tenderloin, thinly sliced
- 2 tablespoons olive oil
- 3 cloves garlic, minced
- 1 tablespoon fresh ginger, grated
- 3 cups snow peas, trimmed
- 1 red bell pepper, thinly sliced
- 1/4 cup low-sodium soy sauce
- 1 tablespoon honey
- 1 tablespoon sesame oil
- 1 tablespoon cornstarch mixed with 2 tablespoons water
- 1 tablespoon sesame seeds (optional)

Instructions:

1. Heat 1 tablespoon of olive oil in a large skillet or wok over medium-high heat.
2. Add the pork slices and stir-fry for 3-4 minutes until browned. Remove from the skillet and set aside.
3. In the same skillet, add the remaining olive oil, garlic, and ginger. Stir-fry for 1-2 minutes until fragrant.
4. Add the snow peas and red bell pepper. Stir-fry for 4-5 minutes until tender-crisp.
5. Return the pork to the skillet.
6. In a small bowl, mix the soy sauce, honey, sesame oil, and cornstarch mixture. Pour over the pork and vegetables.
7. Stir-fry for another 2-3 minutes until the sauce thickens and everything is well coated.
8. Garnish with sesame seeds, if using, and serve immediately.

Nutrition Info per Serving (Serves 4):

- Calories: 300
- Protein: 28g
- Carbohydrates: 15g
- Fiber: 3g
- Sugars: 7g
- Fat: 15g
- Saturated Fat: 3g

Cooking Time:

- **Total: 20 minutes**

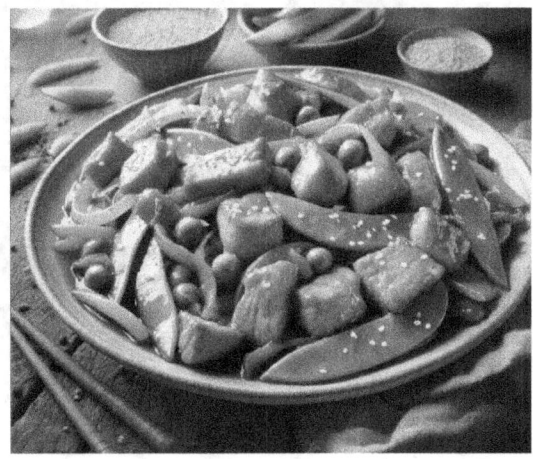

12. Beef and Squash Stew

Ingredients:

- 1 pound beef stew meat, cubed
- 2 tablespoons olive oil
- 1 onion, chopped
- 3 cloves garlic, minced
- 3 cups butternut squash, peeled and cubed
- 2 carrots, peeled and sliced
- 4 cups low-sodium beef broth
- 1 teaspoon dried thyme
- 1 teaspoon dried rosemary
- Fresh parsley for garnish

Instructions:

1. In a large pot, heat olive oil over medium heat. Add the beef and brown on all sides, about 5-7 minutes.
2. Add the onion and garlic, and cook for 3-4 minutes until softened.
3. Stir in the butternut squash, carrots, beef broth, thyme, and rosemary.
4. Bring to a boil, then reduce heat and simmer for 45-50 minutes, until the vegetables are tender and the beef is cooked through.
5. Garnish with fresh parsley before serving.

Nutrition Info per Serving (Serves 6):

- Calories: 280
- Protein: 25g
- Carbohydrates: 20g
- Fiber: 4g
- Sugars: 5g
- Fat: 12g
- Saturated Fat: 3g

Cooking Time:

- **Total: 1 hour**

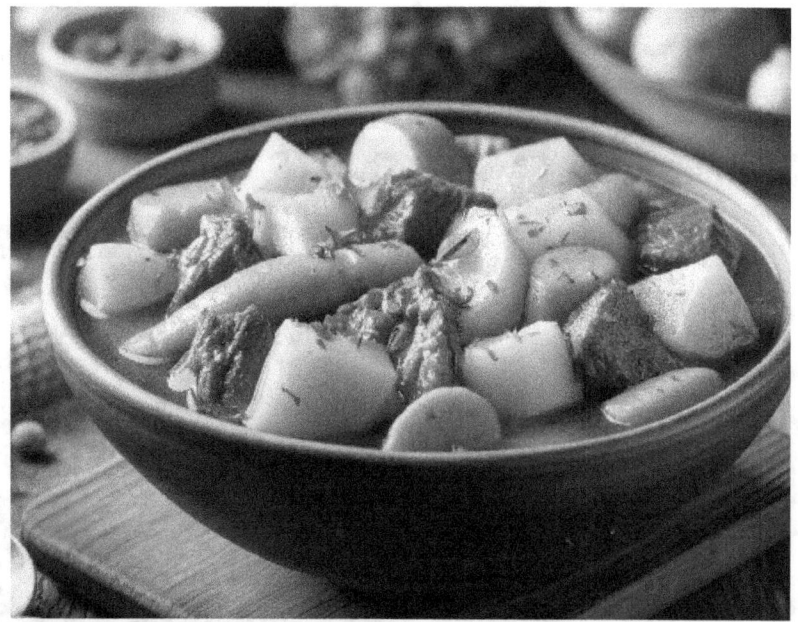

13. Roast Lamb with Rosemary and Garlic

Ingredients:

- 1 boneless leg of lamb (about 3 pounds)
- 4 cloves garlic, minced
- 2 tablespoons fresh rosemary, chopped
- 2 tablespoons olive oil
- 1 lemon, sliced

Instructions:

1. Preheat the oven to 375°F (190°C).
2. In a small bowl, mix the garlic, rosemary, and olive oil.
3. Rub the mixture all over the lamb.
4. Place the lamb in a roasting pan and arrange the lemon slices on top.
5. Roast for 1 hour and 15 minutes, or until the internal temperature reaches 145°F (63°C) for medium-rare.
6. Let rest for 10 minutes before slicing and serving.

Nutrition Info per Serving (Serves 6):

- Calories: 350
- Protein: 28g
- Carbohydrates: 2g
- Fiber: 0.5g
- Sugars: 0.5g
- Fat: 25g
- Saturated Fat: 10g

Cooking Time:

- **Total: 1 hour 30 minutes**

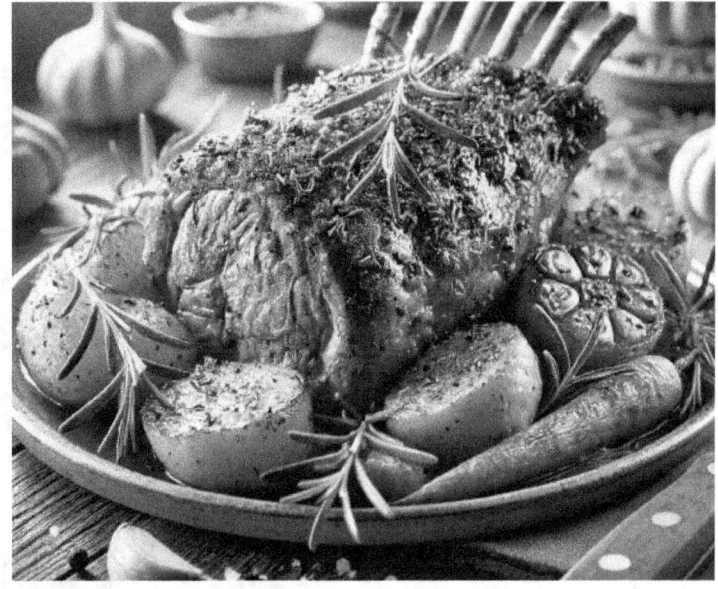

14. Lamb Tagine with Apricots

Ingredients:

- 1 pound lamb shoulder, cubed
- 2 tablespoons olive oil
- 1 onion, chopped
- 3 cloves garlic, minced
- 1 teaspoon ground cinnamon
- 1 teaspoon ground cumin
- 1 teaspoon ground coriander
- 1/2 teaspoon ground turmeric
- 1 cup dried apricots, halved
- 4 cups low-sodium chicken broth
- Fresh cilantro for garnish

Instructions:

1. In a large pot, heat olive oil over medium heat. Add the lamb and brown on all sides, about 5-7 minutes.
2. Add the onion and garlic, and cook for 3-4 minutes until softened.
3. Stir in the cinnamon, cumin, coriander, and turmeric, and cook for another 1-2 minutes.
4. Add the dried apricots and chicken broth, and bring to a boil.
5. Reduce heat and simmer for 1 hour, until the lamb is tender.
6. Garnish with fresh cilantro before serving.

Nutrition Info per Serving (Serves 4):

- Calories: 350
- Protein: 25g
- Carbohydrates: 25g
- Fiber: 5g
- Sugars: 15g
- Fat: 15g
- Saturated Fat: 4g

Cooking Time:

- **Total: 1 hour 15 minutes**

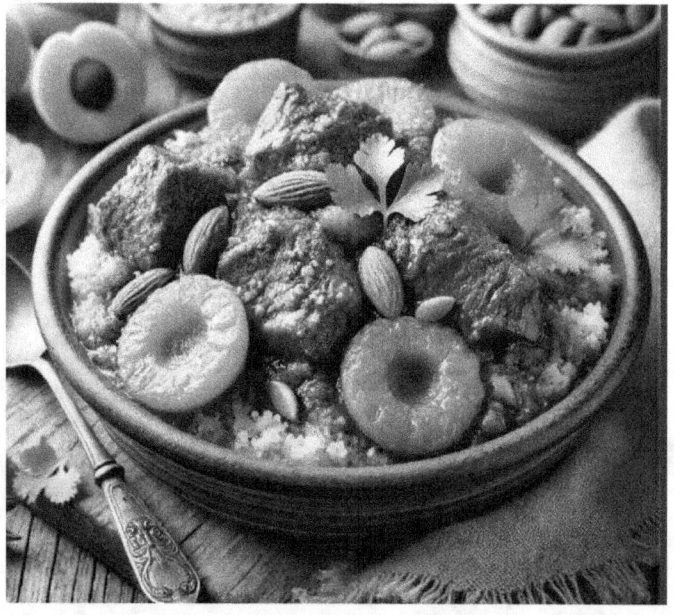

15. Grilled Beef Salad with Arugula

Ingredients:

- 1 pound beef sirloin, thinly sliced
- 2 tablespoons olive oil
- 3 cloves garlic, minced
- 1 teaspoon dried oregano
- 4 cups arugula
- 1 cup cherry tomatoes, halved
- 1/2 red onion, thinly sliced
- 1/4 cup balsamic vinegar
- 2 tablespoons olive oil

Instructions:

1. Preheat the grill to medium-high heat.
2. In a small bowl, mix 2 tablespoons of olive oil, garlic, and oregano. Brush over the beef slices.
3. Grill the beef slices for 3-4 minutes on each side, until cooked to desired doneness. Let cool slightly.
4. In a large bowl, combine the arugula, cherry tomatoes, and red onion.
5. In a small bowl, whisk together the balsamic vinegar and 2 tablespoons olive oil. Pour over the salad and toss to coat.
6. Top the salad with the grilled beef slices and serve immediately.

Nutrition Info per Serving (Serves 4):

- Calories: 320
- Protein: 30g
- Carbohydrates: 10g
- Fiber: 3g
- Sugars: 5g
- Fat: 18g
- Saturated Fat: 4g

Cooking Time:

- **Total: 20 minutes**

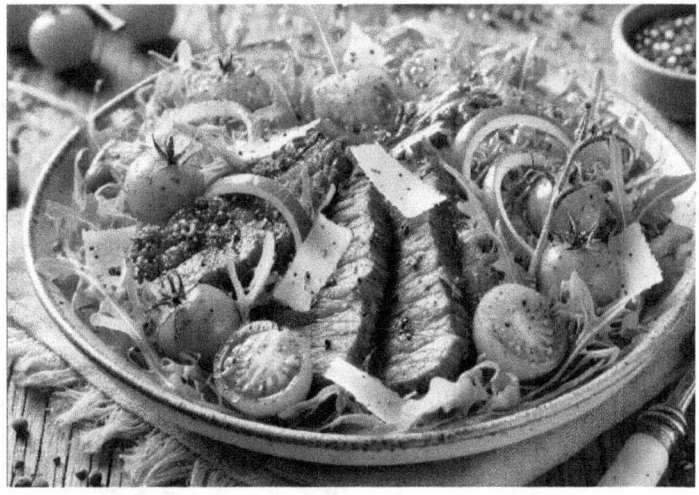

16. Lamb Stir Fry with Zucchini

Ingredients:

- 1 pound lamb loin, thinly sliced
- 2 tablespoons olive oil
- 3 cloves garlic, minced
- 1 tablespoon fresh ginger, grated
- 2 medium zucchinis, sliced
- 1 red bell pepper, sliced
- 1/4 cup low-sodium soy sauce
- 1 tablespoon honey
- 1 tablespoon sesame oil
- 1 tablespoon cornstarch mixed with 2 tablespoons water
- 1 tablespoon sesame seeds (optional)

Instructions:

1. Heat 1 tablespoon of olive oil in a large skillet or wok over medium-high heat.
2. Add the lamb slices and stir-fry for 3-4 minutes until browned. Remove from the skillet and set aside.
3. In the same skillet, add the remaining olive oil, garlic, and ginger. Stir-fry for 1-2 minutes until fragrant.
4. Add the zucchini and red bell pepper. Stir-fry for 4-5 minutes until tender-crisp.
5. Return the lamb to the skillet.
6. In a small bowl, mix the soy sauce, honey, sesame oil, and cornstarch mixture. Pour over the lamb and vegetables.
7. Stir-fry for another 2-3 minutes until the sauce thickens and everything is well coated.
8. Garnish with sesame seeds, if using, and serve immediately.

Nutrition Info per Serving (Serves 4):

- Calories: 320
- Protein: 28g
- Carbohydrates: 15g
- Fiber: 3g
- Sugars: 6g
- Fat: 18g
- Saturated Fat: 6g

Cooking Time:

- **Total: 20 minutes**

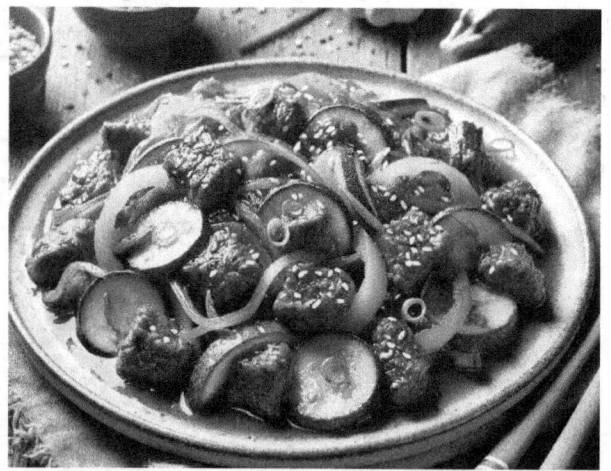

17. Beef and Broccoli Quinoa Bowl

Ingredients:

- 1 pound beef sirloin, thinly sliced
- 1 cup quinoa, rinsed
- 2 cups broccoli florets
- 2 tablespoons olive oil
- 3 cloves garlic, minced
- 1/4 cup low-sodium soy sauce
- 1 tablespoon honey
- 1 tablespoon sesame oil
- 1 tablespoon cornstarch mixed with 2 tablespoons water
- 1 tablespoon sesame seeds (optional)

Instructions:

1. Cook quinoa according to package instructions. Set aside.
2. Heat 1 tablespoon of olive oil in a large skillet over medium-high heat.
3. Add the beef slices and stir-fry for 3-4 minutes until browned. Remove from the skillet and set aside.
4. In the same skillet, add the remaining olive oil and garlic. Stir-fry for 1-2 minutes until fragrant.
5. Add the broccoli florets and stir-fry for 4-5 minutes until tender-crisp.
6. Return the beef to the skillet.
7. In a small bowl, mix the soy sauce, honey, sesame oil, and cornstarch mixture. Pour over the beef and broccoli.
8. Stir-fry for another 2-3 minutes until the sauce thickens and everything is well coated.
9. Serve the beef and broccoli over quinoa, garnished with sesame seeds, if using.

Nutrition Info per Serving (Serves 4):

- Calories: 370
- Protein: 30g
- Carbohydrates: 35g
- Fiber: 5g
- Sugars: 7g
- Fat: 14g
- Saturated Fat: 3.5g

Cooking Time:

- Total: 30 minutes

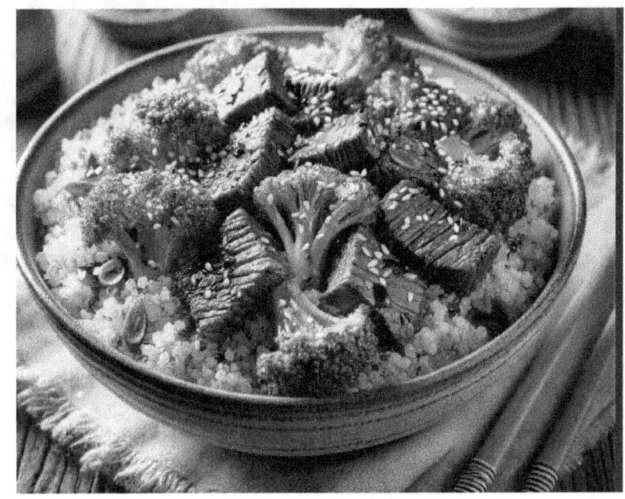

18. Lamb Chops with Cauliflower Rice

Ingredients:

- 8 lamb chops
- 2 tablespoons olive oil
- 3 cloves garlic, minced
- 1 teaspoon dried rosemary
- 1 large head of cauliflower, riced
- 1/4 cup fresh parsley, chopped

Instructions:

1. Preheat the grill to medium-high heat.
2. In a small bowl, mix 2 tablespoons of olive oil, garlic, and rosemary. Brush over the lamb chops.
3. Grill the lamb chops for 4-5 minutes on each side, or until desired doneness. Let rest for 5 minutes.
4. While the lamb chops are grilling, heat a large skillet over medium heat and add the riced cauliflower. Cook for 5-7 minutes until tender.
5. Stir in the chopped parsley.
6. Serve the lamb chops with the cauliflower rice.

Nutrition Info per Serving (Serves 4):

- Calories: 420
- Protein: 32g
- Carbohydrates: 10g
- Fiber: 4g
- Sugars: 3g
- Fat: 28g
- Saturated Fat: 10g

Cooking Time:

- **Total: 25 minutes**

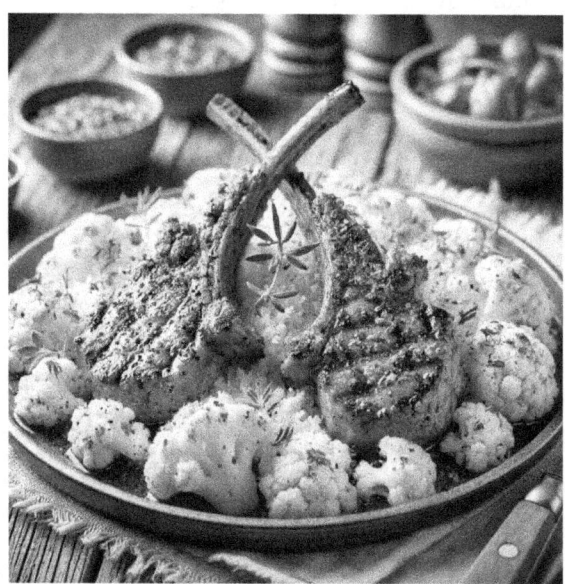

19. Lamb Salad with Mixed Greens

Ingredients:

- 1 pound lamb loin, thinly sliced
- 2 tablespoons olive oil
- 3 cloves garlic, minced
- 1 teaspoon dried oregano
- 4 cups mixed greens (arugula, spinach, kale)
- 1 cup cherry tomatoes, halved
- 1/2 red onion, thinly sliced
- 1/4 cup balsamic vinegar
- 2 tablespoons olive oil

Instructions:

1. Heat 1 tablespoon of olive oil in a large skillet over medium-high heat.
2. Add the lamb slices and garlic, and cook for 3-4 minutes until browned. Remove from heat and let cool slightly.
3. In a large bowl, combine the mixed greens, cherry tomatoes, and red onion.
4. In a small bowl, whisk together the balsamic vinegar and 2 tablespoons olive oil. Pour over the salad and toss to coat.
5. Top the salad with the cooked lamb slices and serve immediately.

Nutrition Info per Serving (Serves 4):

- Calories: 320
- Protein: 30g
- Carbohydrates: 10g
- Fiber: 3g
- Sugars: 5g
- Fat: 18g
- Saturated Fat: 6g

Cooking Time:

- **Total: 20 minutes**

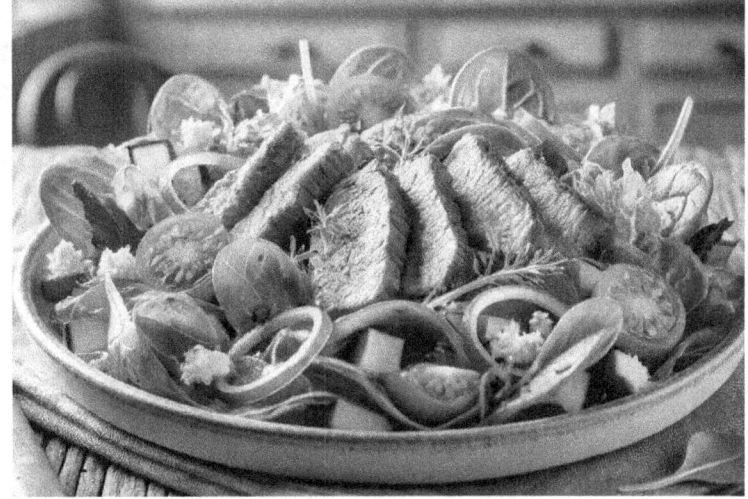

20. Beef Tomato Stew

Ingredients:

- 1 pound beef stew meat, cubed
- 2 tablespoons olive oil
- 1 onion, chopped
- 3 cloves garlic, minced
- 3 large tomatoes, chopped
- 2 carrots, peeled and sliced
- 2 celery stalks, sliced
- 4 cups low-sodium beef broth
- 1 teaspoon dried thyme
- Fresh parsley for garnish

Instructions:

1. In a large pot, heat olive oil over medium heat. Add the beef and brown on all sides, about 5-7 minutes.
2. Add the onion and garlic, and cook for 3-4 minutes until softened.
3. Stir in the tomatoes, carrots, celery, beef broth, and thyme.
4. Bring to a boil, then reduce heat and simmer for 1 hour, until the beef is tender.
5. Garnish with fresh parsley before serving.

Nutrition Info per Serving (Serves 6):

- Calories: 280
- Protein: 25g
- Carbohydrates: 15g
- Fiber: 4g
- Sugars: 7g
- Fat: 12g
- Saturated Fat: 4g

Cooking Time:

- **Total: 1 hour 15 minutes**

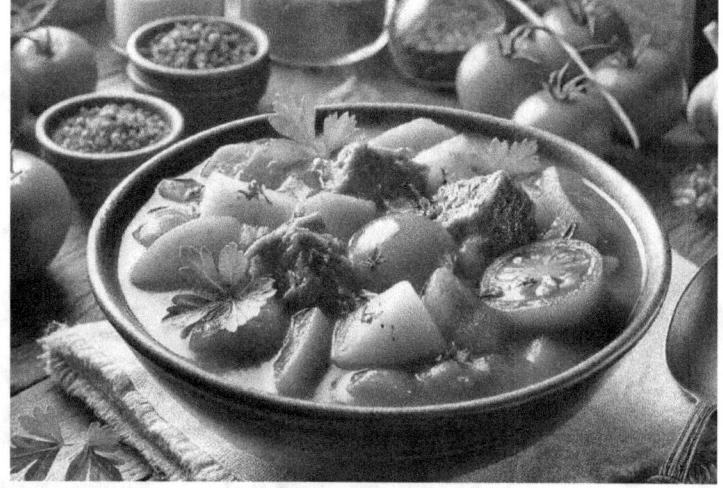

21. Beef and Green Bean Salad

Ingredients:

- 1 pound beef sirloin, thinly sliced
- 2 tablespoons olive oil
- 3 cloves garlic, minced
- 1 teaspoon dried oregano
- 4 cups green beans, trimmed and blanched
- 1/2 red onion, thinly sliced
- 1/4 cup balsamic vinegar
- 2 tablespoons olive oil

Instructions:

1. Heat 1 tablespoon of olive oil in a large skillet over medium-high heat.
2. Add the beef slices and garlic, and cook for 3-4 minutes until browned. Remove from heat and let cool slightly.
3. In a large bowl, combine the green beans and red onion.
4. In a small bowl, whisk together the balsamic vinegar and 2 tablespoons olive oil. Pour over the green beans and toss to coat.
5. Top the salad with the cooked beef slices and serve immediately.

Nutrition Info per Serving (Serves 4):

- Calories: 300
- Protein: 28g
- Carbohydrates: 12g
- Fiber: 4g
- Sugars: 5g
- Fat: 16g
- Saturated Fat: 4g

Cooking Time:

- **Total: 20 minutes**

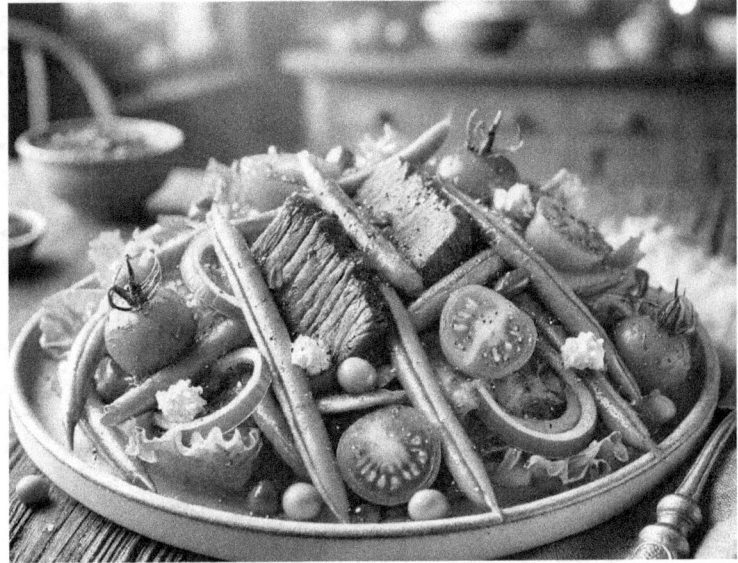

22. Pork Tenderloin with Cherry Sauce

Ingredients:

- 1 pork tenderloin (about 1 pound)
- 2 tablespoons olive oil
- 1/2 cup fresh or frozen cherries, pitted
- 1/4 cup balsamic vinegar
- 1 tablespoon honey
- 1 teaspoon dried thyme

Instructions:

1. Preheat the oven to 375°F (190°C).
2. In a small bowl, mix 1 tablespoon of olive oil and thyme. Rub over the pork tenderloin.
3. Heat the remaining olive oil in a large ovenproof skillet over medium-high heat. Brown the pork tenderloin on all sides, about 5 minutes.
4. Transfer the skillet to the oven and roast for 20-25 minutes, until the internal temperature reaches 145°F (63°C).
5. While the pork is roasting, combine the cherries, balsamic vinegar, and honey in a small saucepan. Bring to a simmer and cook for 10-12 minutes, until the sauce is thickened.
6. Let the pork rest for 5 minutes before slicing and serving with the cherry sauce.

Nutrition Info per Serving (Serves 4):

- Calories: 250
- Protein: 24g
- Carbohydrates: 15g
- Fiber: 2g
- Sugars: 10g
- Fat: 12g
- Saturated Fat: 3g

Cooking Time:

- **Total: 35 minutes**

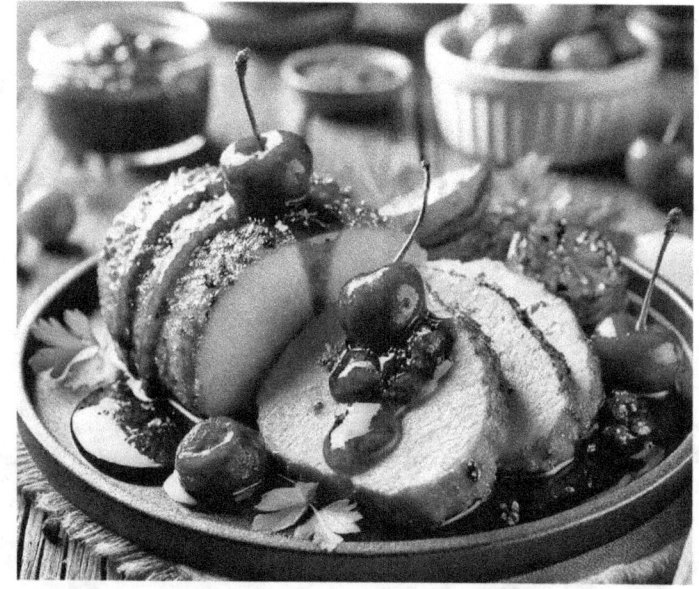

23. Lamb Loin with Pomegranate Sauce

Ingredients:

- 1 pound lamb loin
- 2 tablespoons olive oil
- 1/2 cup pomegranate juice
- 1/4 cup chicken broth, low sodium
- 1 tablespoon honey
- 1 teaspoon dried thyme
- Fresh pomegranate seeds for garnish

Instructions:

1. Preheat the oven to 375°F (190°C).
2. In a small bowl, mix 1 tablespoon of olive oil and thyme. Rub over the lamb loin.
3. Heat the remaining olive oil in a large ovenproof skillet over medium-high heat. Brown the lamb loin on all sides, about 5 minutes.
4. Transfer the skillet to the oven and roast for 20-25 minutes, until the internal temperature reaches 145°F (63°C).
5. While the lamb is roasting, combine the pomegranate juice, chicken broth, and honey in a small saucepan. Bring to a simmer and cook for 10-12 minutes, until the sauce is thickened.
6. Let the lamb rest for 5 minutes before slicing and serving with the pomegranate sauce. Garnish with fresh pomegranate seeds.

Nutrition Info per Serving (Serves 4):

- Calories: 320
- Protein: 28g
- Carbohydrates: 15g
- Fiber: 1g
- Sugars: 12g
- Fat: 18g
- Saturated Fat: 6g

Cooking Time:

- **Total: 35 minutes**

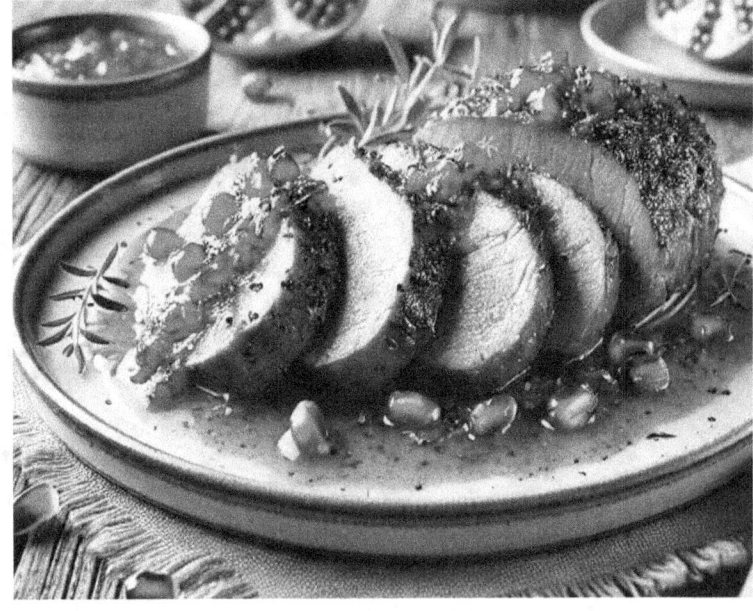

Fish & Seafood Recipes

1. Grilled Salmon with Dill and Lemon

Ingredients:

- 4 salmon fillets (6 oz each)
- 2 tablespoons olive oil
- 2 cloves garlic, minced
- 2 tablespoons fresh dill, chopped
- 1 lemon, sliced
- 1 lemon, juiced

Instructions:

1. Preheat the grill to medium-high heat.
2. In a small bowl, mix the olive oil, garlic, dill, and lemon juice.
3. Brush the mixture over the salmon fillets.
4. Place the salmon fillets on the grill, skin-side down. Place lemon slices on top.
5. Grill for 4-6 minutes per side, or until the salmon is cooked through and flakes easily with a fork.
6. Serve immediately.

Nutrition Info per Serving (Serves 4):

- Calories: 350
- Protein: 35g
- Carbohydrates: 2g
- Fiber: 0.5g
- Sugars: 1g
- Fat: 22g
- Saturated Fat: 4g

Cooking Time:

- **Total: 15 minutes**

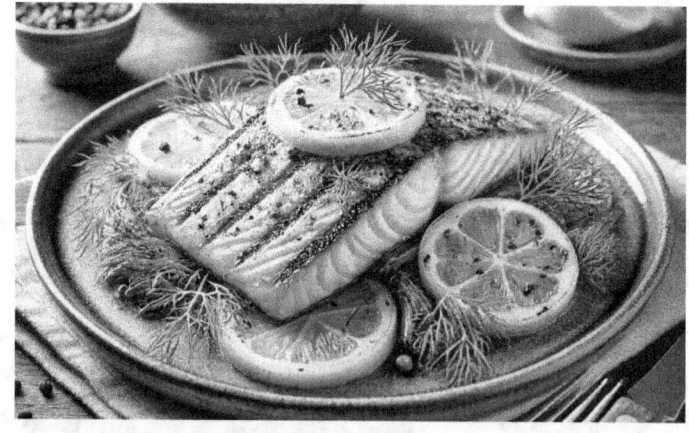

2. Baked Cod with Parsley Pesto

Ingredients:

- 4 cod fillets (6 oz each)
- 2 tablespoons olive oil
- 1 cup fresh parsley, chopped
- 1/4 cup pine nuts
- 2 cloves garlic, minced
- 1/4 cup olive oil (for pesto)
- 1 lemon, juiced

Instructions:

1. Preheat the oven to 375°F (190°C).
2. In a food processor, combine the parsley, pine nuts, garlic, 1/4 cup olive oil, and lemon juice. Blend until smooth to make the parsley pesto.
3. Place the cod fillets in a baking dish and brush with 2 tablespoons of olive oil.
4. Spread the parsley pesto evenly over the cod fillets.
5. Bake for 20-25 minutes, or until the fish is opaque and flakes easily with a fork.
6. Serve immediately.

Nutrition Info per Serving (Serves 4):

- Calories: 310
- Protein: 32g
- Carbohydrates: 4g
- Fiber: 1g
- Sugars: 0.5g
- Fat: 18g
- Saturated Fat: 2.5g

Cooking Time:

- **Total: 30 minutes**

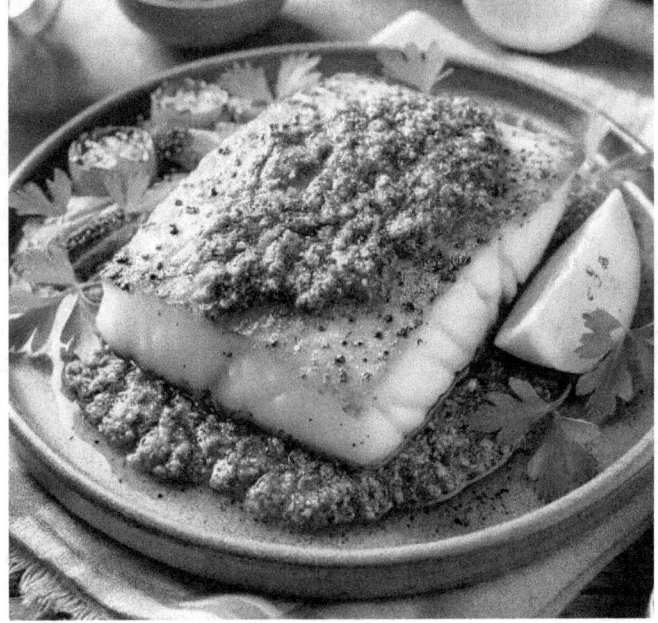

3. Seared Scallops with Cauliflower Puree

Ingredients:

- 1 pound sea scallops
- 2 tablespoons olive oil
- 1 large cauliflower, chopped
- 1 cup low-sodium chicken broth
- 2 cloves garlic, minced
- 1 tablespoon fresh thyme, chopped
- 1 tablespoon lemon juice
- Fresh parsley for garnish

Instructions:

1. In a large pot, bring the cauliflower and chicken broth to a boil. Reduce heat and simmer for 10-15 minutes until the cauliflower is tender.
2. Use an immersion blender to puree the cauliflower until smooth. Stir in garlic and thyme. Keep warm.
3. Pat the scallops dry and season with lemon juice.
4. Heat olive oil in a large skillet over medium-high heat.
5. Sear the scallops for 2-3 minutes on each side, until golden brown and cooked through.
6. Serve the scallops on top of the cauliflower puree, garnished with fresh parsley.

Nutrition Info per Serving (Serves 4):

- Calories: 260
- Protein: 25g
- Carbohydrates: 12g
- Fiber: 4g
- Sugars: 3g
- Fat: 12g
- Saturated Fat: 1.5g

Cooking Time:

- **Total: 25 minutes**

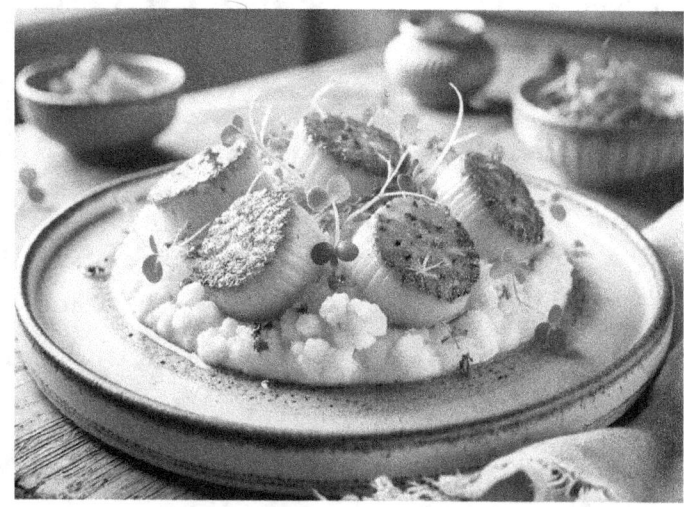

4. Mackerel in Tomato Sauce

Ingredients:

- 4 mackerel fillets (6 oz each)
- 2 tablespoons olive oil
- 1 onion, chopped
- 2 cloves garlic, minced
- 1 can (14.5 oz) diced tomatoes, no salt added
- 1 teaspoon dried oregano
- 1 teaspoon dried basil
- 1/4 cup fresh parsley, chopped

Instructions:

1. Preheat the oven to 375°F (190°C).
2. Heat olive oil in a large skillet over medium heat. Add the onion and garlic, and cook for 3-4 minutes until softened.
3. Stir in the diced tomatoes, oregano, and basil. Simmer for 10 minutes until the sauce thickens.
4. Place the mackerel fillets in a baking dish and pour the tomato sauce over them.
5. Bake for 20-25 minutes, or until the mackerel is cooked through and flakes easily with a fork.
6. Garnish with fresh parsley and serve immediately.

Nutrition Info per Serving (Serves 4):

- Calories: 330
- Protein: 30g
- Carbohydrates: 8g
- Fiber: 2g
- Sugars: 4g
- Fat: 20g
- Saturated Fat: 4g

Cooking Time:

- **Total: 35 minutes**

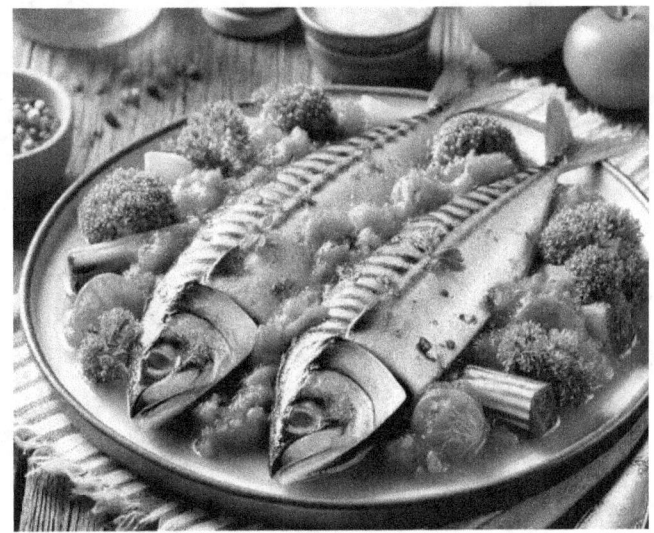

5. Clam Soup with Vegetables

Ingredients:

- 2 tablespoons olive oil
- 1 onion, chopped
- 3 cloves garlic, minced
- 2 carrots, peeled and sliced
- 2 celery stalks, sliced
- 1 zucchini, diced
- 1 cup low-sodium chicken broth
- 1 cup water
- 2 pounds clams, scrubbed and cleaned
- 1 teaspoon dried thyme
- Fresh parsley for garnish

Instructions:

1. Heat olive oil in a large pot over medium heat. Add the onion and garlic, and cook for 3-4 minutes until softened.
2. Add the carrots, celery, and zucchini. Cook for another 5-7 minutes until the vegetables are tender.
3. Pour in the chicken broth and water, and bring to a boil.
4. Add the clams and dried thyme. Cover and cook for 5-7 minutes until the clams open. Discard any that do not open.
5. Garnish with fresh parsley and serve immediately.

Nutrition Info per Serving (Serves 4):

- Calories: 220
- Protein: 22g
- Carbohydrates: 12g
- Fiber: 3g
- Sugars: 4g
- Fat: 10g
- Saturated Fat: 1.5g

Cooking Time:

- **Total: 25 minutes**

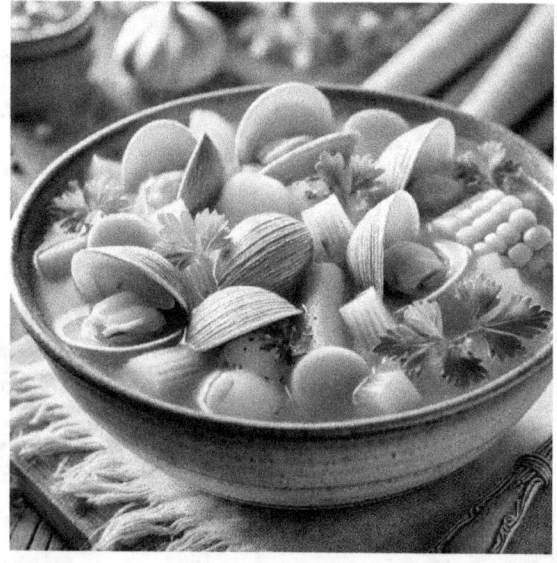

6. Grilled Tuna Steaks with Avocado Salsa

Ingredients:

- 4 tuna steaks (6 oz each)
- 2 tablespoons olive oil
- 1 teaspoon dried oregano
- 2 avocados, diced
- 1 small red onion, finely chopped
- 1 jalapeno, seeded and minced
- 1/4 cup fresh cilantro, chopped
- 2 tablespoons lime juice

Instructions:

1. Preheat the grill to medium-high heat.
2. Brush the tuna steaks with olive oil and sprinkle with oregano.
3. Grill the tuna steaks for 3-4 minutes on each side, or until desired doneness.
4. In a medium bowl, combine the diced avocados, red onion, jalapeno, cilantro, and lime juice.
5. Serve the tuna steaks topped with the avocado salsa.

Nutrition Info per Serving (Serves 4):

- Calories: 400
- Protein: 35g
- Carbohydrates: 10g
- Fiber: 7g
- Sugars: 1g
- Fat: 26g
- Saturated Fat: 4g

Cooking Time:

- **Total: 15 minutes**

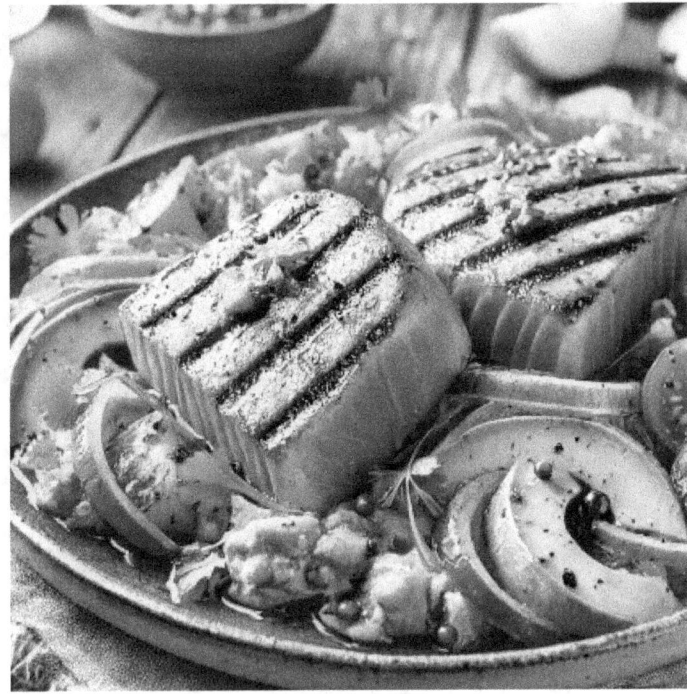

7. Poached Halibut with Dill Sauce

Ingredients:

- 4 halibut fillets (6 oz each)
- 4 cups low-sodium chicken broth
- 1 lemon, sliced
- 1/4 cup fresh dill, chopped
- 1 cup plain Greek yogurt
- 1 tablespoon lemon juice
- 1 tablespoon olive oil

Instructions:

1. In a large pot, bring the chicken broth and lemon slices to a simmer.
2. Add the halibut fillets and poach for 8-10 minutes, until the fish is opaque and flakes easily with a fork.
3. While the fish is poaching, mix the Greek yogurt, fresh dill, lemon juice, and olive oil in a small bowl to make the dill sauce.
4. Remove the halibut fillets from the broth and serve with the dill sauce.

Nutrition Info per Serving (Serves 4):

- Calories: 300
- Protein: 35g
- Carbohydrates: 5g
- Fiber: 0.5g
- Sugars: 3g
- Fat: 15g
- Saturated Fat: 3g

Cooking Time:

- **Total: 15 minutes**

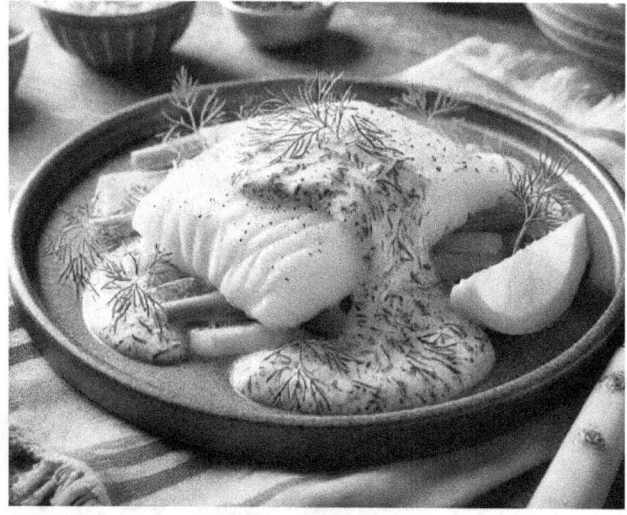

8. Shrimp Ceviche with Lime and Cilantro

Ingredients:

- 1 pound raw shrimp, peeled, deveined, and chopped
- 1/2 cup lime juice
- 1/4 cup lemon juice
- 1 small red onion, finely chopped
- 1 jalapeno, seeded and minced
- 1 cup cherry tomatoes, halved
- 1/4 cup fresh cilantro, chopped
- 1 avocado, diced

Instructions:

1. In a large bowl, combine the chopped shrimp, lime juice, and lemon juice. Cover and refrigerate for 1 hour until the shrimp is opaque and fully cooked.
2. Drain the shrimp and mix in the red onion, jalapeno, cherry tomatoes, cilantro, and avocado.
3. Serve immediately.

Nutrition Info per Serving (Serves 4):

- Calories: 220
- Protein: 25g
- Carbohydrates: 10g
- Fiber: 5g
- Sugars: 3g
- Fat: 10g
- Saturated Fat: 1.5g

Cooking Time:

- **Total: 1 hour 15 minutes (including refrigeration time)**

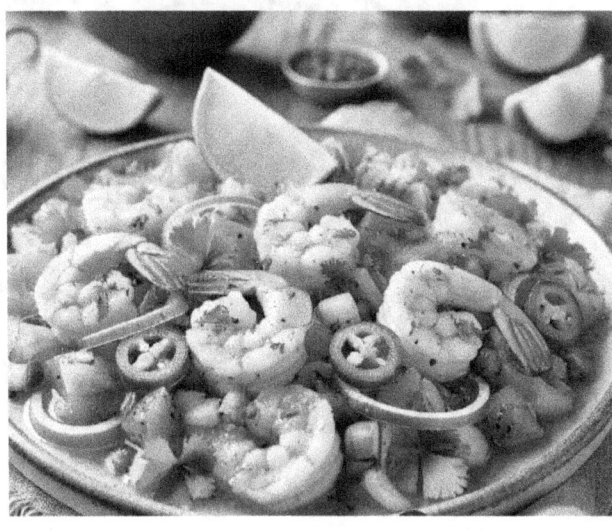

9. Salmon and Spinach Salad

Ingredients:

- 4 salmon fillets (6 oz each)
- 2 tablespoons olive oil
- 1 teaspoon dried thyme
- 6 cups baby spinach
- 1 cup cherry tomatoes, halved
- 1/2 red onion, thinly sliced
- 1/4 cup balsamic vinegar
- 2 tablespoons olive oil (for dressing)
- 1 tablespoon Dijon mustard

Instructions:

1. Preheat the oven to 375°F (190°C).
2. Brush the salmon fillets with olive oil and sprinkle with thyme.
3. Bake the salmon fillets for 15-20 minutes, or until the salmon is cooked through and flakes easily with a fork.
4. In a large bowl, combine the baby spinach, cherry tomatoes, and red onion.
5. In a small bowl, whisk together the balsamic vinegar, 2 tablespoons olive oil, and Dijon mustard to make the dressing.
6. Top the salad with the baked salmon fillets and drizzle with the dressing before serving.

Nutrition Info per Serving (Serves 4):

- Calories: 350
- Protein: 35g
- Carbohydrates: 8g
- Fiber: 2g
- Sugars: 5g
- Fat: 20g
- Saturated Fat: 3g

Cooking Time:

- **Total: 25 minutes**

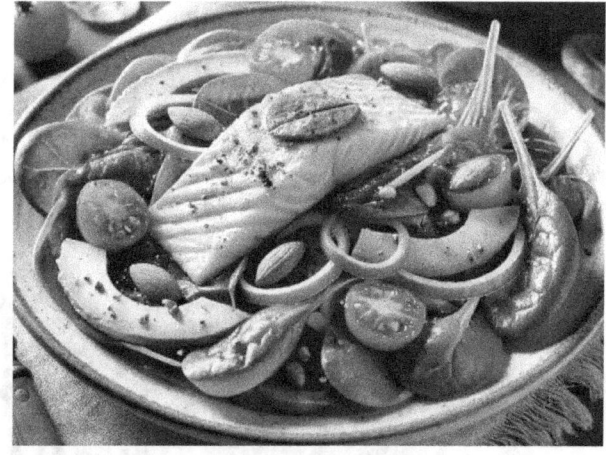

10. Lobster Salad with Mixed Greens
Ingredients:
- 2 lobster tails, cooked and chopped
- 4 cups mixed greens (arugula, spinach, kale)
- 1 avocado, diced
- 1 cup cherry tomatoes, halved
- 1/4 cup fresh chives, chopped
- 1/4 cup olive oil
- 2 tablespoons lemon juice
- 1 teaspoon Dijon mustard

Instructions:
1. In a large bowl, combine the mixed greens, avocado, cherry tomatoes, and fresh chives.
2. In a small bowl, whisk together the olive oil, lemon juice, and Dijon mustard to make the dressing.
3. Add the chopped lobster tails to the salad and drizzle with the dressing.
4. Toss gently to combine and serve immediately.

Nutrition Info per Serving (Serves 4):
- Calories: 300
- Protein: 18g
- Carbohydrates: 10g
- Fiber: 5g
- Sugars: 3g
- Fat: 22g
- Saturated Fat: 3.5g

Cooking Time:
- **Total: 20 minutes**

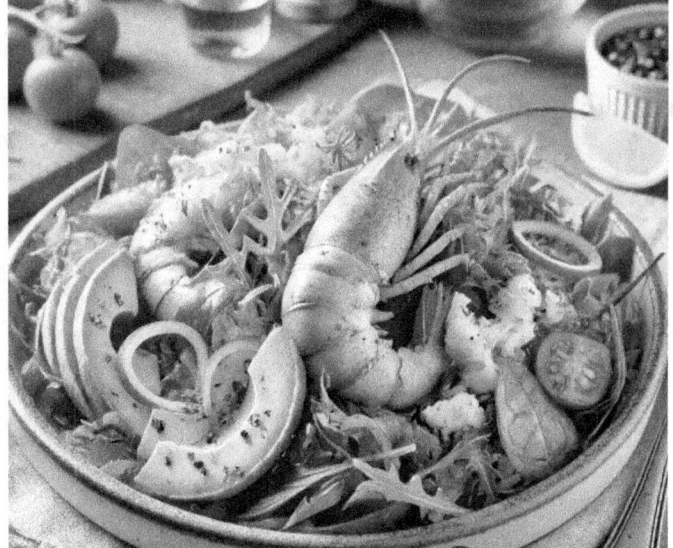

11. Baked Trout with Almonds

Ingredients:

- 4 trout fillets (6 oz each)
- 2 tablespoons olive oil
- 1/2 cup sliced almonds
- 2 cloves garlic, minced
- 1 tablespoon lemon juice
- 1 tablespoon fresh parsley, chopped

Instructions:

1. Preheat the oven to 375°F (190°C).
2. Place the trout fillets in a baking dish and brush with olive oil.
3. Sprinkle the minced garlic and sliced almonds evenly over the trout.
4. Bake for 15-20 minutes, until the fish is cooked through and flakes easily with a fork.
5. Drizzle with lemon juice and garnish with fresh parsley before serving.

Nutrition Info per Serving (Serves 4):

- Calories: 320
- Protein: 35g
- Carbohydrates: 4g
- Fiber: 2g
- Sugars: 0.5g
- Fat: 18g
- Saturated Fat: 3g

Cooking Time:

- **Total: 20 minutes**

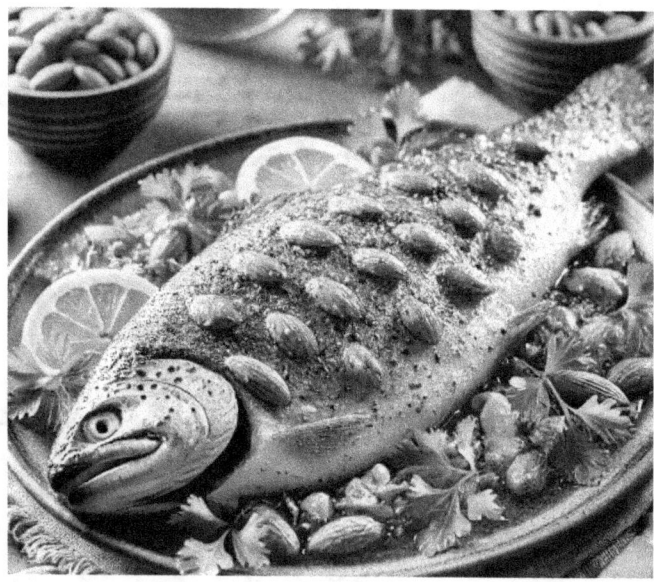

12. Halibut Stir-Fry with Bell Peppers

Ingredients:

- 4 halibut fillets (6 oz each), cut into bite-sized pieces
- 2 tablespoons olive oil
- 1 red bell pepper, sliced
- 1 yellow bell pepper, sliced
- 1 green bell pepper, sliced
- 3 cloves garlic, minced
- 1 tablespoon fresh ginger, grated
- 1/4 cup low-sodium soy sauce
- 1 tablespoon honey
- 1 tablespoon sesame oil
- 1 tablespoon cornstarch mixed with 2 tablespoons water

Instructions:

1. Heat 1 tablespoon of olive oil in a large skillet or wok over medium-high heat.
2. Add the halibut pieces and cook for 2-3 minutes until browned. Remove from the skillet and set aside.
3. In the same skillet, add the remaining olive oil, garlic, and ginger. Stir-fry for 1-2 minutes until fragrant.
4. Add the bell peppers and stir-fry for 4-5 minutes until tender-crisp.
5. Return the halibut to the skillet.
6. In a small bowl, mix the soy sauce, honey, sesame oil, and cornstarch mixture. Pour over the halibut and vegetables.
7. Stir-fry for another 2-3 minutes until the sauce thickens and everything is well coated.
8. Serve immediately.

Nutrition Info per Serving (Serves 4):

- Calories: 300
- Protein: 35g
- Carbohydrates: 12g
- Fiber: 3g
- Sugars: 6g
- Fat: 12g
- Saturated Fat: 2g

Cooking Time:

- **Total: 20 minutes**

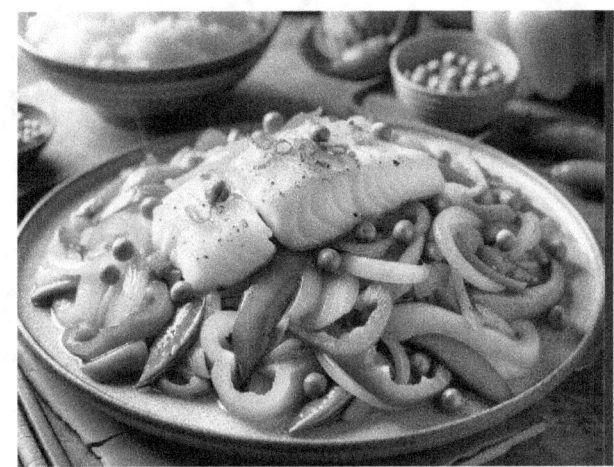

13. Tilapia with Mango Salsa

Ingredients:

- 4 tilapia fillets (6 oz each)
- 2 tablespoons olive oil
- 2 mangos, peeled and diced
- 1 small red onion, finely chopped
- 1 jalapeno, seeded and minced
- 1/4 cup fresh cilantro, chopped
- 2 tablespoons lime juice

Instructions:

1. Preheat the oven to 375°F (190°C).
2. Brush the tilapia fillets with olive oil and place them in a baking dish.
3. Bake for 15-20 minutes, until the fish is opaque and flakes easily with a fork.
4. While the fish is baking, combine the diced mangos, red onion, jalapeno, cilantro, and lime juice in a medium bowl.
5. Serve the tilapia topped with the mango salsa.

Nutrition Info per Serving (Serves 4):

- Calories: 320
- Protein: 30g
- Carbohydrates: 20g
- Fiber: 4g
- Sugars: 15g
- Fat: 12g
- Saturated Fat: 2g

Cooking Time:

- **Total: 20 minutes**

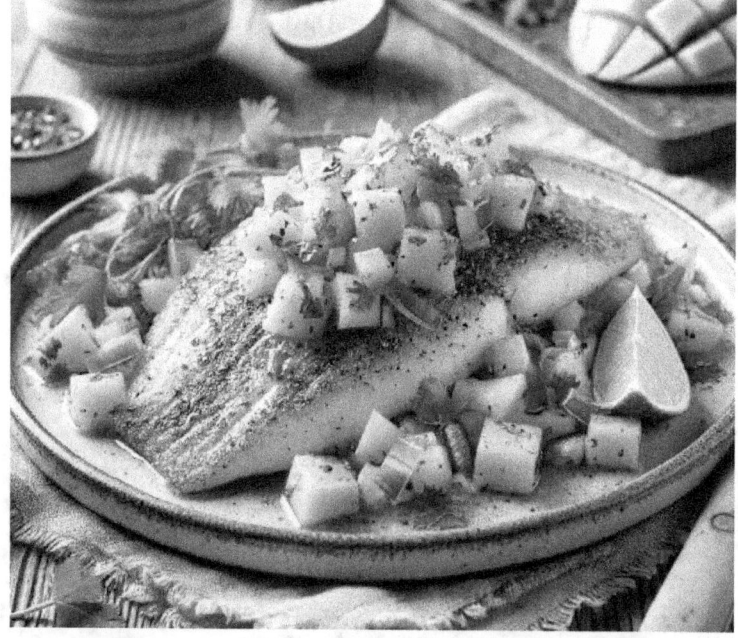

14. Oysters on the Half Shell with Mignonette Sauce

Ingredients:

- 12 fresh oysters, shucked
- 1/4 cup red wine vinegar
- 1 tablespoon shallots, finely chopped
- 1 tablespoon fresh parsley, finely chopped
- 1/2 teaspoon freshly ground black pepper

Instructions:

1. Arrange the shucked oysters on a serving platter.
2. In a small bowl, mix together the red wine vinegar, shallots, parsley, and black pepper.
3. Spoon a small amount of the mignonette sauce over each oyster.
4. Serve immediately.

Nutrition Info per Serving (Serves 4):

- Calories: 70
- Protein: 6g
- Carbohydrates: 3g
- Fiber: 0g
- Sugars: 0g
- Fat: 3g
- Saturated Fat: 0.5g

Cooking Time:

- **Total: 15 minutes**

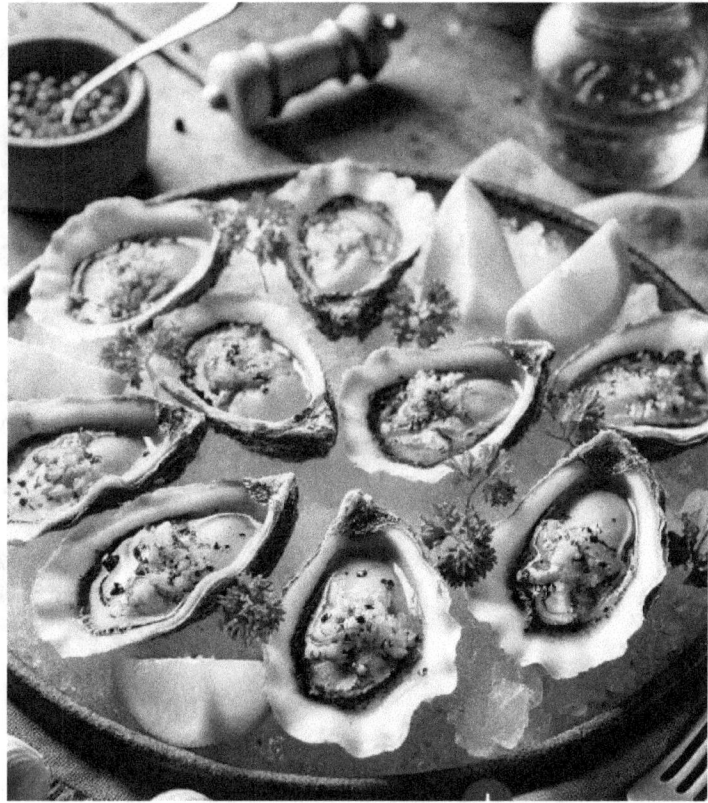

15. Grilled Swordfish with Basil Oil

Ingredients:

- 4 swordfish steaks (6 oz each)
- 2 tablespoons olive oil
- 1/2 cup fresh basil leaves
- 2 cloves garlic, minced
- 1/4 cup olive oil (for basil oil)
- 1 tablespoon lemon juice

Instructions:

1. Preheat the grill to medium-high heat.
2. Brush the swordfish steaks with 2 tablespoons of olive oil.
3. Grill the swordfish steaks for 4-5 minutes on each side, or until cooked through.
4. In a blender, combine the basil leaves, garlic, 1/4 cup olive oil, and lemon juice. Blend until smooth to make the basil oil.
5. Serve the grilled swordfish topped with the basil oil.

Nutrition Info per Serving (Serves 4):

- Calories: 400
- Protein: 35g
- Carbohydrates: 2g
- Fiber: 0.5g
- Sugars: 0.5g
- Fat: 28g
- Saturated Fat: 6g

Cooking Time:

- **Total: 15 minutes**

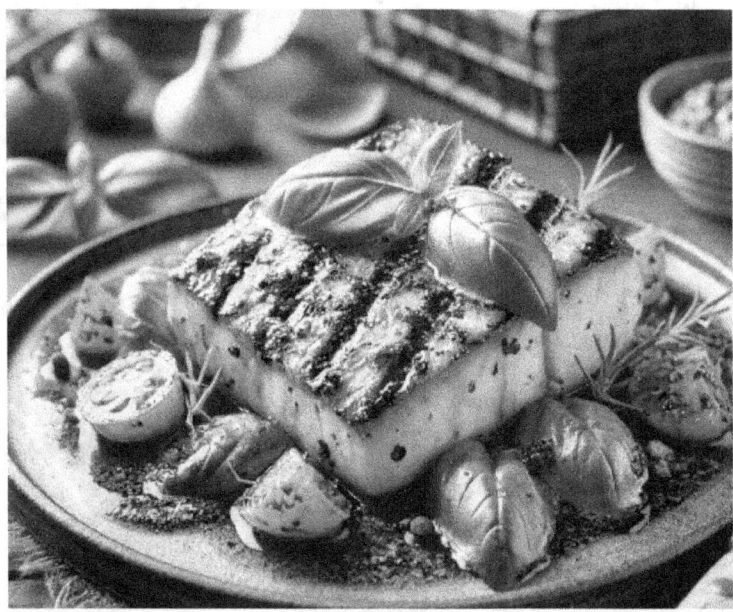

16. Flounder with Herb Crust

Ingredients:

- 4 flounder fillets (6 oz each)
- 1/2 cup almond flour
- 1/4 cup fresh parsley, chopped
- 1/4 cup fresh basil, chopped
- 2 cloves garlic, minced
- 1 lemon, zested and juiced
- 2 tablespoons olive oil

Instructions:

1. Preheat the oven to 375°F (190°C).
2. In a bowl, mix the almond flour, parsley, basil, garlic, lemon zest, and half of the lemon juice.
3. Brush the flounder fillets with olive oil.
4. Press the herb mixture onto the top of each fillet.
5. Place the fillets on a baking sheet and bake for 15-20 minutes, or until the fish is cooked through and flakes easily with a fork.
6. Drizzle with the remaining lemon juice before serving.

Nutrition Info per Serving (Serves 4):

- Calories: 320
- Protein: 32g
- Carbohydrates: 6g
- Fiber: 2g
- Sugars: 1g
- Fat: 20g
- Saturated Fat: 3g

Cooking Time:

- **Total: 25 minutes**

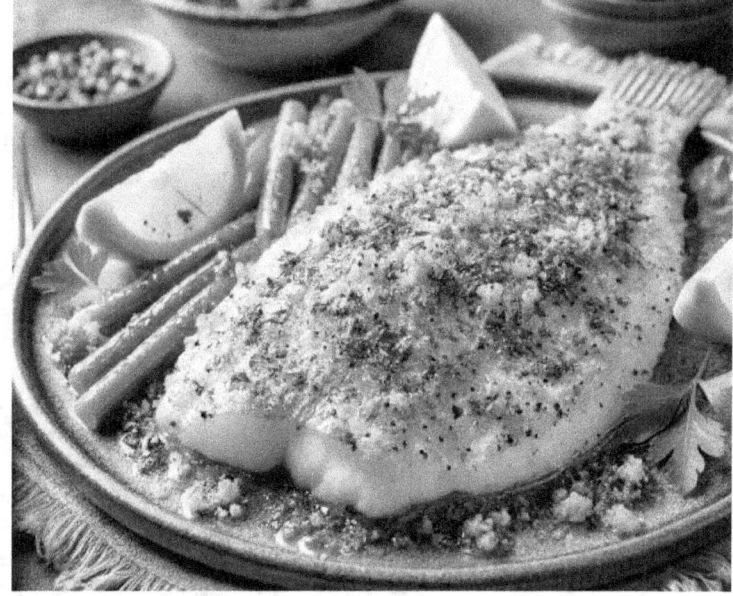

17. Sea Bass with Fennel and Orange

Ingredients:

- 4 sea bass fillets (6 oz each)
- 2 tablespoons olive oil
- 1 fennel bulb, thinly sliced
- 1 orange, thinly sliced
- 1 tablespoon fresh thyme
- 1/4 cup orange juice

Instructions:

1. Preheat the oven to 375°F (190°C).
2. Heat 1 tablespoon of olive oil in a large ovenproof skillet over medium heat.
3. Add the fennel slices and cook for 5-7 minutes, until softened.
4. Place the sea bass fillets on top of the fennel, and arrange the orange slices over the fish.
5. Sprinkle with fresh thyme and drizzle with the remaining olive oil and orange juice.
6. Transfer the skillet to the oven and bake for 15-20 minutes, or until the fish is opaque and flakes easily with a fork.
7. Serve immediately.

Nutrition Info per Serving (Serves 4):

- Calories: 280
- Protein: 28g
- Carbohydrates: 10g
- Fiber: 3g
- Sugars: 6g
- Fat: 14g
- Saturated Fat: 2g

Cooking Time:

- **Total: 25 minutes**

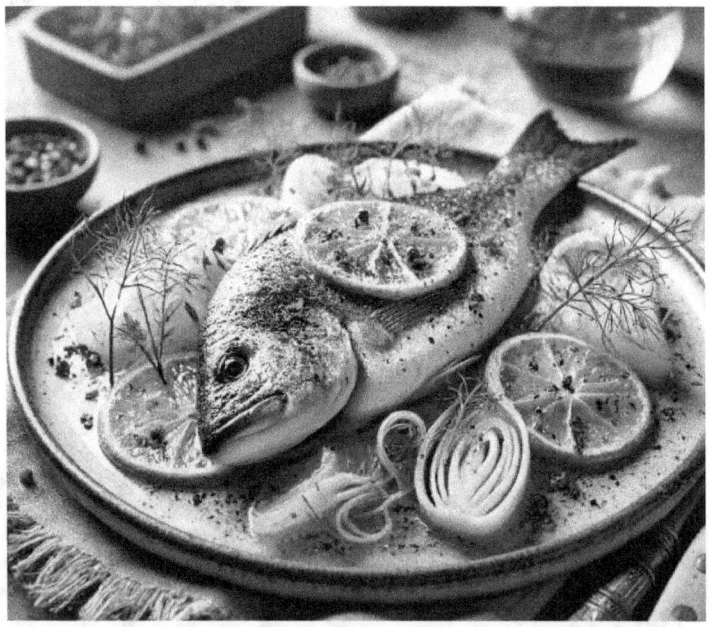

18. Canned Tuna Salad with Olives and Tomatoes

Ingredients:

- 2 cans (5 oz each) tuna in water, drained
- 1 cup cherry tomatoes, halved
- 1/2 cup Kalamata olives, pitted and sliced
- 1/4 cup red onion, finely chopped
- 2 tablespoons fresh parsley, chopped
- 2 tablespoons olive oil
- 2 tablespoons lemon juice

Instructions:

1. In a large bowl, combine the tuna, cherry tomatoes, olives, red onion, and parsley.
2. In a small bowl, whisk together the olive oil and lemon juice.
3. Pour the dressing over the salad and toss to combine.
4. Serve immediately.

Nutrition Info per Serving (Serves 4):

- Calories: 200
- Protein: 20g
- Carbohydrates: 5g
- Fiber: 2g
- Sugars: 3g
- Fat: 12g
- Saturated Fat: 2g

Cooking Time:

- **Total: 10 minutes**

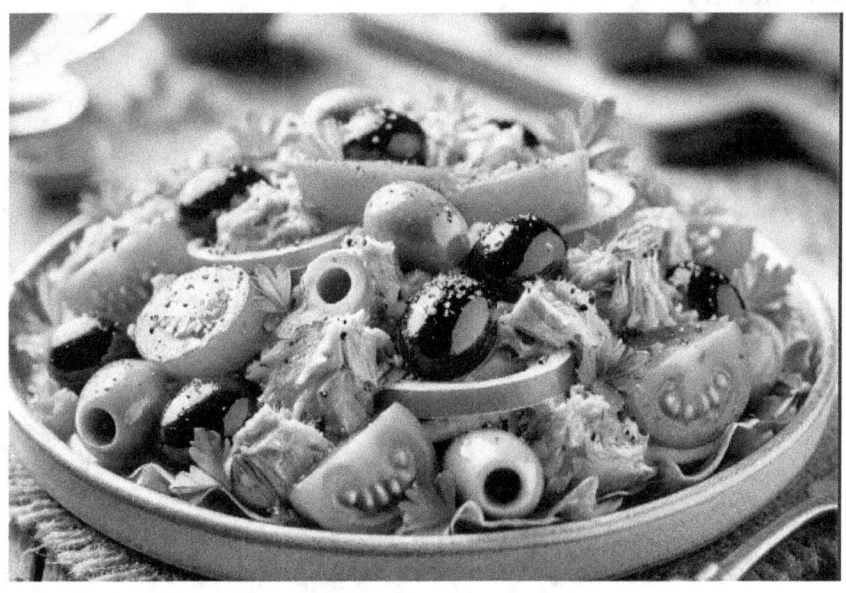

19. Seared Tuna with Sesame Seeds

Ingredients:

- 4 tuna steaks (6 oz each)
- 2 tablespoons olive oil
- 1/4 cup sesame seeds
- 2 tablespoons soy sauce (low sodium)
- 1 tablespoon fresh ginger, grated
- 1 tablespoon lime juice

Instructions:

1. In a small bowl, mix the soy sauce, ginger, and lime juice.
2. Brush the tuna steaks with olive oil and dip each steak into the sesame seeds to coat.
3. Heat a non-stick skillet over medium-high heat.
4. Sear the tuna steaks for 1-2 minutes on each side, until the sesame seeds are golden brown and the tuna is cooked to desired doneness.
5. Drizzle with the soy sauce mixture and serve immediately.

Nutrition Info per Serving (Serves 4):

- Calories: 350
- Protein: 40g
- Carbohydrates: 5g
- Fiber: 1g
- Sugars: 1g
- Fat: 18g
- Saturated Fat: 3g

Cooking Time:

- **Total: 10 minutes**

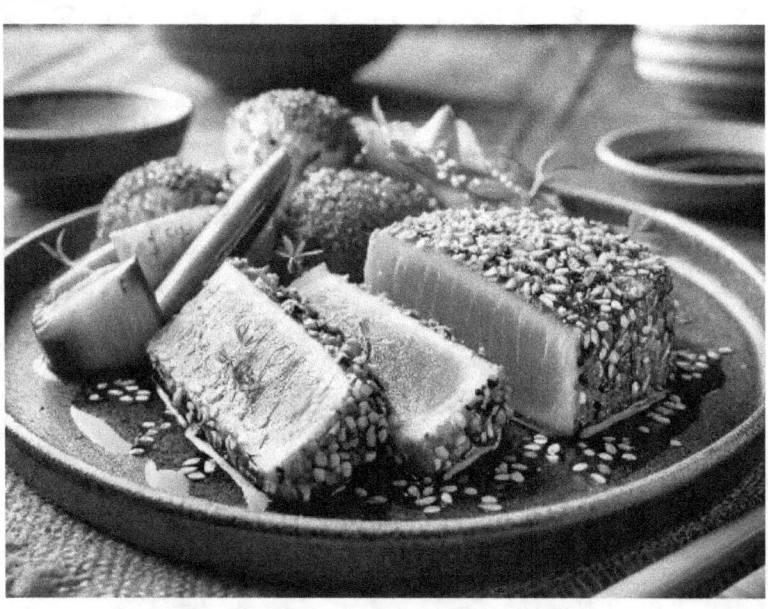

20. Clam and Spinach Pasta

Ingredients:

- 1 pound whole wheat spaghetti
- 2 tablespoons olive oil
- 3 cloves garlic, minced
- 2 cups baby spinach
- 2 pounds clams, scrubbed and cleaned
- 1/2 cup white wine
- 1/4 cup fresh parsley, chopped
- 1 lemon, juiced

Instructions:

1. Cook the spaghetti according to package instructions. Drain and set aside.
2. In a large pot, heat the olive oil over medium heat. Add the garlic and cook for 1-2 minutes until fragrant.
3. Add the baby spinach and cook until wilted, about 2 minutes.
4. Add the clams and white wine, cover, and cook for 5-7 minutes, or until the clams open. Discard any that do not open.
5. Toss the cooked spaghetti with the clam mixture.
6. Drizzle with lemon juice and garnish with fresh parsley before serving.

Nutrition Info per Serving (Serves 4):

- Calories: 400
- Protein: 25g
- Carbohydrates: 55g
- Fiber: 8g
- Sugars: 3g
- Fat: 10g
- Saturated Fat: 1.5g

Cooking Time:

- **Total: 20 minutes**

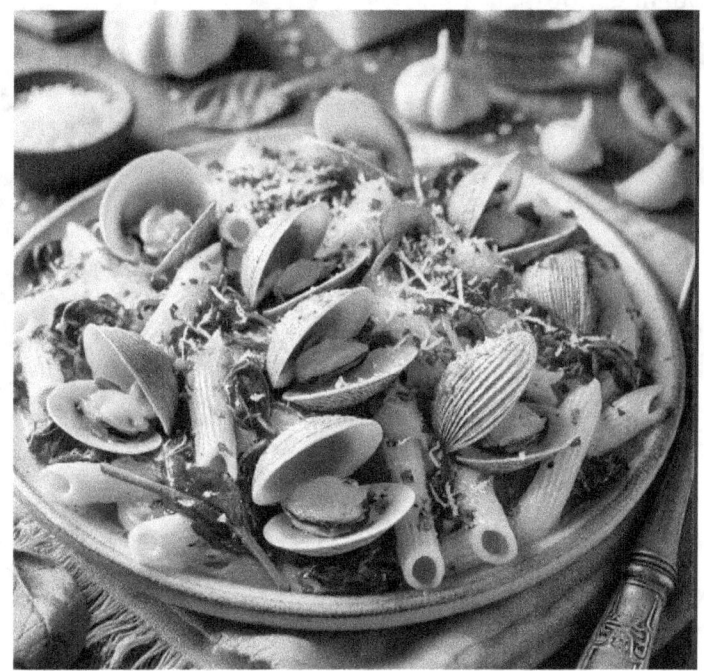

21. Grilled Branzino with Lemon Butter

Ingredients:

- 4 branzino fillets (6 oz each)
- 2 tablespoons olive oil
- 1 lemon, sliced
- 1/4 cup unsalted butter, melted
- 1 tablespoon fresh parsley, chopped

Instructions:

1. Preheat the grill to medium-high heat.
2. Brush the branzino fillets with olive oil.
3. Grill the fillets for 4-5 minutes on each side, or until the fish is opaque and flakes easily with a fork.
4. In a small bowl, mix the melted butter with the juice of half the lemon and the parsley.
5. Serve the grilled branzino drizzled with lemon butter and garnished with lemon slices.

Nutrition Info per Serving (Serves 4):

- Calories: 350
- Protein: 30g
- Carbohydrates: 2g
- Fiber: 0.5g
- Sugars: 0.5g
- Fat: 24g
- Saturated Fat: 9g

Cooking Time:

- **Total: 15 minutes**

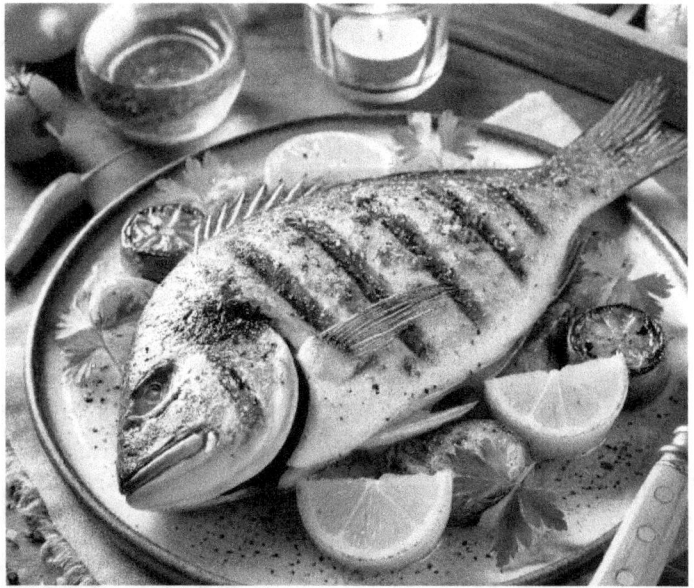

22. Anchovy and Green Bean Salad

Ingredients:

- 1 pound green beans, trimmed and blanched
- 1 can (2 oz) anchovy fillets, drained and chopped
- 1/2 cup cherry tomatoes, halved
- 1/4 cup Kalamata olives, pitted and sliced
- 2 tablespoons fresh parsley, chopped
- 2 tablespoons olive oil
- 1 tablespoon red wine vinegar

Instructions:

1. In a large bowl, combine the blanched green beans, anchovies, cherry tomatoes, olives, and parsley.
2. In a small bowl, whisk together the olive oil and red wine vinegar.
3. Pour the dressing over the salad and toss to combine.
4. Serve immediately.

Nutrition Info per Serving (Serves 4):

- Calories: 150
- Protein: 6g
- Carbohydrates: 10g
- Fiber: 4g
- Sugars: 3g
- Fat: 10g
- Saturated Fat: 2g

Cooking Time:

- **Total: 15 minutes**

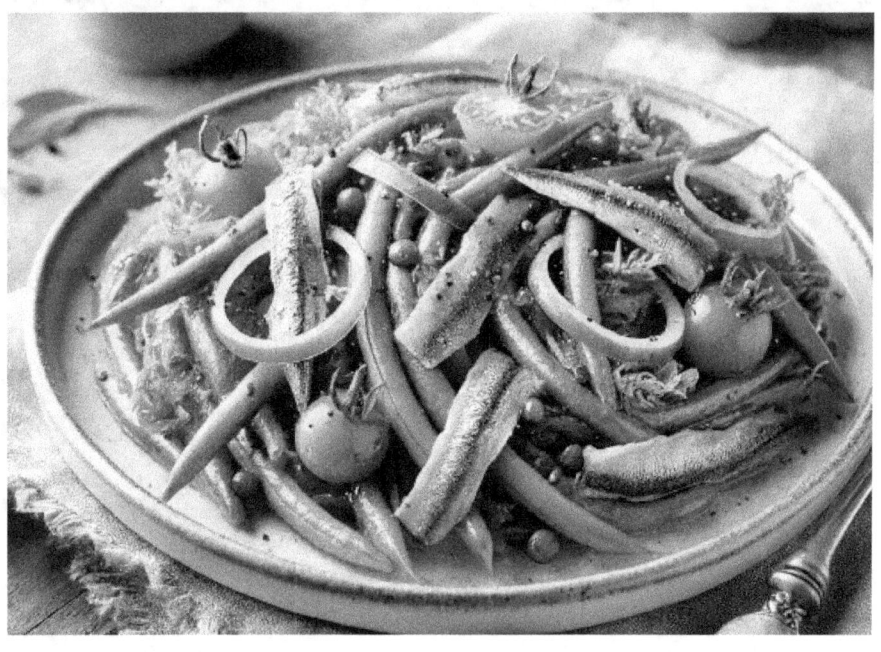

23. Monkfish with Tomato and Capers
Ingredients:
- 4 monkfish fillets (6 oz each)
- 2 tablespoons olive oil
- 1 onion, chopped
- 3 cloves garlic, minced
- 1 can (14.5 oz) diced tomatoes, no salt added
- 1/4 cup capers, rinsed
- 1 tablespoon fresh oregano, chopped
- 1 lemon, juiced

Instructions:
1. Preheat the oven to 375°F (190°C).
2. Heat the olive oil in a large ovenproof skillet over medium heat. Add the onion and garlic, and cook for 3-4 minutes until softened.
3. Stir in the diced tomatoes, capers, and oregano.
4. Place the monkfish fillets in the skillet, spooning some of the tomato mixture over the top.
5. Transfer the skillet to the oven and bake for 15-20 minutes, or until the fish is opaque and flakes easily with a fork.
6. Drizzle with lemon juice before serving.

Nutrition Info per Serving (Serves 4):
- Calories: 300
- Protein: 28g
- Carbohydrates: 10g
- Fiber: 3g
- Sugars: 5g
- Fat: 14g
- Saturated Fat: 2g

Cooking Time:
- **Total: 25 minutes**

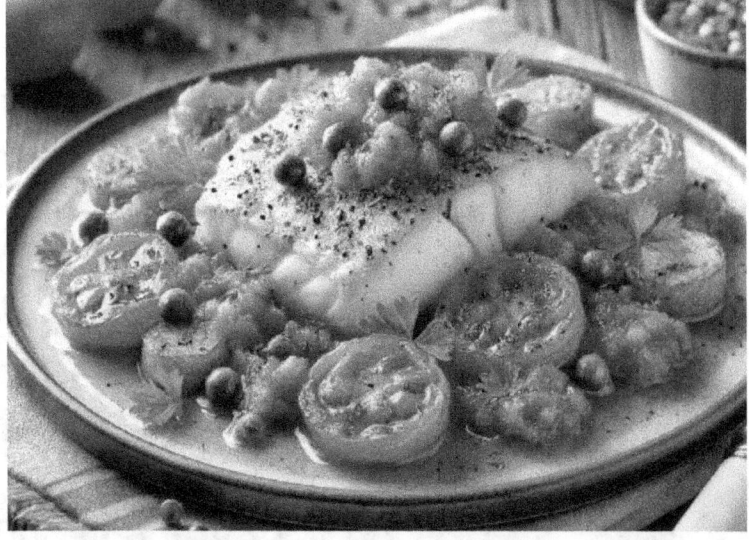

Soup & Stew Recipes

1. Lentil Soup with Kale

Ingredients:

- 1 cup dried lentils, rinsed
- 2 tablespoons olive oil
- 1 onion, chopped
- 3 cloves garlic, minced
- 3 carrots, peeled and sliced
- 2 celery stalks, sliced
- 6 cups low-sodium vegetable broth
- 1 teaspoon dried thyme
- 1 teaspoon dried oregano
- 4 cups chopped kale, stems removed
- 1 lemon, juiced

Instructions:

1. In a large pot, heat the olive oil over medium heat. Add the onion and garlic, and cook for 3-4 minutes until softened.
2. Add the carrots and celery, and cook for another 5 minutes.
3. Stir in the lentils, vegetable broth, thyme, and oregano. Bring to a boil.
4. Reduce heat and simmer for 25-30 minutes, or until the lentils are tender.
5. Stir in the chopped kale and cook for another 5 minutes until wilted.
6. Add lemon juice before serving.

Nutrition Info per Serving (Serves 6):

- Calories: 220
- Protein: 10g
- Carbohydrates: 30g
- Fiber: 10g
- Sugars: 6g
- Fat: 7g
- Saturated Fat: 1g

Cooking Time:

- **Total: 45 minutes**

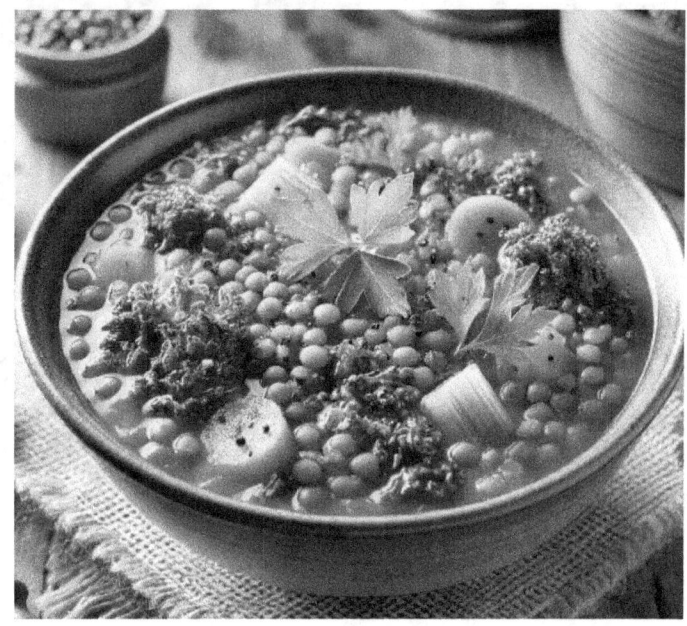

2. Beef Bone Broth

Ingredients:

- 2 pounds beef bones (marrow bones, knuckles, oxtails)
- 1 onion, quartered
- 2 carrots, chopped
- 2 celery stalks, chopped
- 3 cloves garlic, smashed
- 1 tablespoon apple cider vinegar
- 10 cups water
- 2 bay leaves
- 1 teaspoon dried thyme

Instructions:

1. Preheat the oven to 400°F (200°C). Place the beef bones on a baking sheet and roast for 30 minutes.
2. Transfer the roasted bones to a large pot. Add the onion, carrots, celery, garlic, apple cider vinegar, water, bay leaves, and thyme.
3. Bring to a boil, then reduce heat and simmer for 12-24 hours, skimming foam and fat occasionally.
4. Strain the broth through a fine-mesh sieve and discard the solids.
5. Let cool before refrigerating or freezing.

Nutrition Info per Serving (Serves 8):

- Calories: 100
- Protein: 6g
- Carbohydrates: 3g
- Fiber: 1g
- Sugars: 1g
- Fat: 6g
- Saturated Fat: 2g

Cooking Time:

- **Total: 12-24 hours**

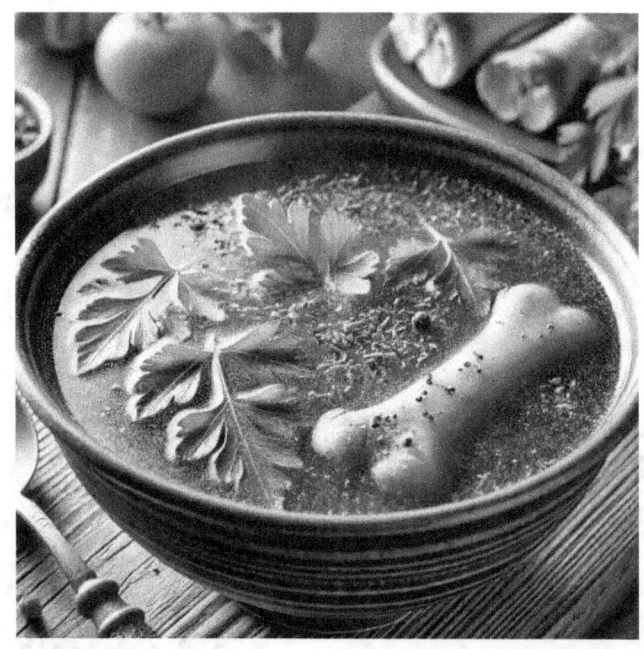

3. Miso Soup with Tofu and Seaweed

Ingredients:

- 6 cups water
- 1/4 cup miso paste
- 1 cup tofu, cubed
- 1/4 cup dried seaweed (wakame), rehydrated
- 2 green onions, sliced

Instructions:

1. In a medium pot, bring the water to a simmer over medium heat.
2. In a small bowl, dissolve the miso paste in a little warm water, then add it to the pot.
3. Add the tofu cubes and rehydrated seaweed to the pot. Simmer for 5 minutes.
4. Garnish with sliced green onions before serving.

Nutrition Info per Serving (Serves 4):

- Calories: 80
- Protein: 6g
- Carbohydrates: 8g
- Fiber: 2g
- Sugars: 2g
- Fat: 3g
- Saturated Fat: 0.5g

Cooking Time:

- **Total: 10 minutes**

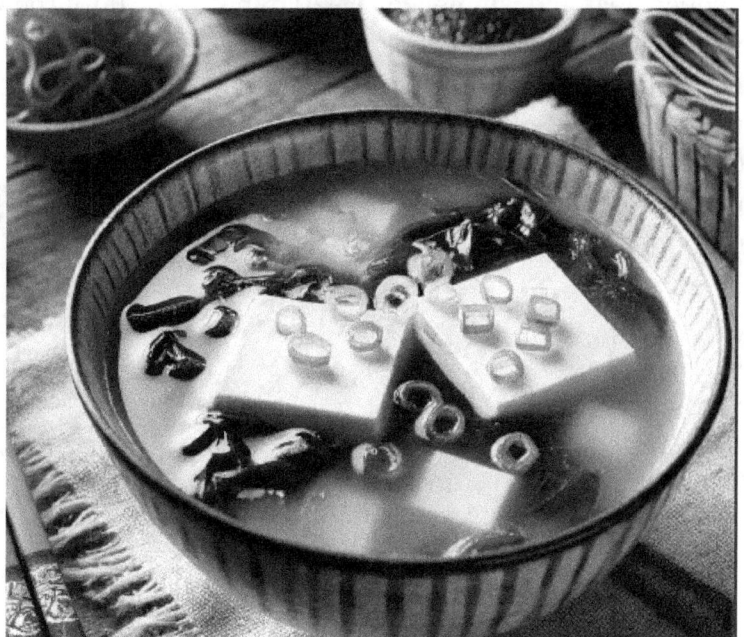

4. Spinach and White Bean Soup

Ingredients:

- 2 tablespoons olive oil
- 1 onion, chopped
- 3 cloves garlic, minced
- 2 carrots, peeled and sliced
- 2 celery stalks, sliced
- 4 cups low-sodium vegetable broth
- 1 can (15 oz) white beans, drained and rinsed
- 4 cups fresh spinach
- 1 teaspoon dried thyme
- 1 teaspoon dried oregano
- 1 lemon, juiced

Instructions:

1. In a large pot, heat the olive oil over medium heat. Add the onion and garlic, and cook for 3-4 minutes until softened.
2. Add the carrots and celery, and cook for another 5 minutes.
3. Stir in the vegetable broth, white beans, thyme, and oregano. Bring to a boil.
4. Reduce heat and simmer for 15-20 minutes, or until the vegetables are tender.
5. Stir in the spinach and cook for another 2-3 minutes until wilted.
6. Add lemon juice before serving.

Nutrition Info per Serving (Serves 6):

- Calories: 180
- Protein: 7g
- Carbohydrates: 25g
- Fiber: 8g
- Sugars: 4g
- Fat: 7g
- Saturated Fat: 1g

Cooking Time:

- **Total: 35 minutes**

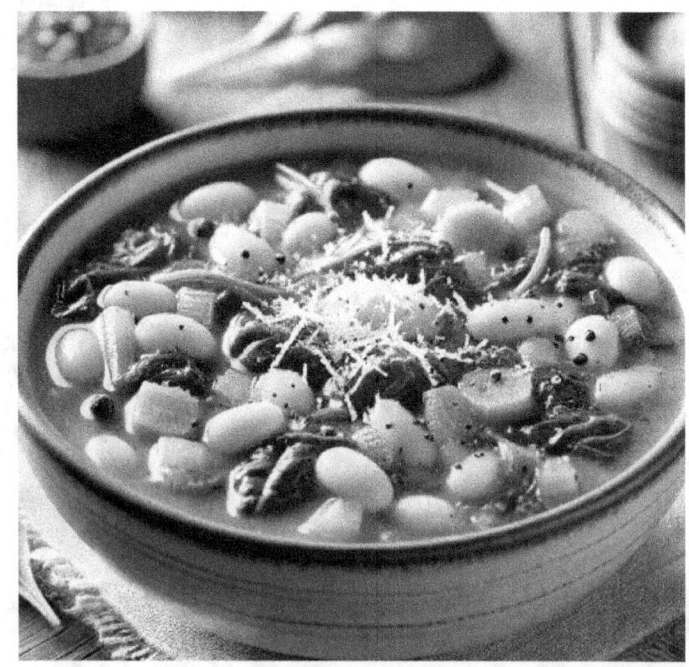

5. Carrot and Coriander Soup

Ingredients:

- 2 tablespoons olive oil
- 1 onion, chopped
- 3 cloves garlic, minced
- 1 teaspoon ground coriander
- 6 large carrots, peeled and chopped
- 4 cups low-sodium vegetable broth
- 1/4 cup fresh cilantro, chopped
- 1 lemon, juiced

Instructions:

1. In a large pot, heat the olive oil over medium heat. Add the onion and garlic, and cook for 3-4 minutes until softened.
2. Stir in the ground coriander and cook for another minute.
3. Add the carrots and vegetable broth. Bring to a boil, then reduce heat and simmer for 20-25 minutes, or until the carrots are tender.
4. Use an immersion blender to puree the soup until smooth.
5. Stir in the fresh cilantro and lemon juice before serving.

Nutrition Info per Serving (Serves 6):

- Calories: 150
- Protein: 2g
- Carbohydrates: 20g
- Fiber: 5g
- Sugars: 10g
- Fat: 7g
- Saturated Fat: 1g

Cooking Time:

- **Total: 35 minutes**

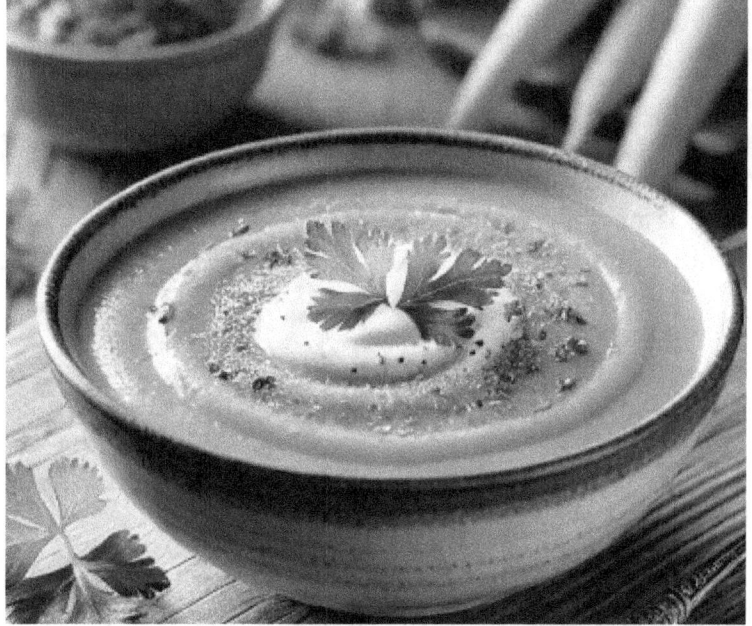

6. Pumpkin Soup with Nutmeg

Ingredients:

- 2 tablespoons olive oil
- 1 onion, chopped
- 3 cloves garlic, minced
- 4 cups pumpkin puree
- 4 cups low-sodium vegetable broth
- 1 teaspoon ground nutmeg
- 1 teaspoon ground cinnamon
- 1 cup coconut milk
- Fresh parsley for garnish

Instructions:

1. In a large pot, heat the olive oil over medium heat. Add the onion and garlic, and cook for 3-4 minutes until softened.
2. Stir in the pumpkin puree, vegetable broth, nutmeg, and cinnamon. Bring to a boil.
3. Reduce heat and simmer for 20 minutes, stirring occasionally.
4. Stir in the coconut milk and cook for another 5 minutes.
5. Use an immersion blender to puree the soup until smooth.
6. Garnish with fresh parsley before serving.

Nutrition Info per Serving (Serves 6):

- Calories: 200
- Protein: 3g
- Carbohydrates: 25g
- Fiber: 6g
- Sugars: 10g
- Fat: 10g
- Saturated Fat: 7g

Cooking Time:

- **Total: 30 minutes**

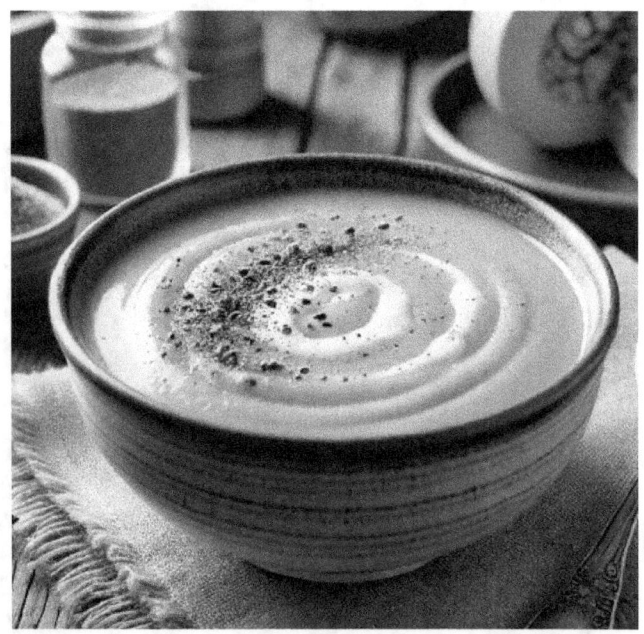

7. Broccoli and Almond Soup

Ingredients:

- 2 tablespoons olive oil
- 1 onion, chopped
- 3 cloves garlic, minced
- 4 cups broccoli florets
- 4 cups low-sodium vegetable broth
- 1/2 cup almond flour
- 1/2 cup unsweetened almond milk
- 1 teaspoon dried thyme
- Fresh chives for garnish

Instructions:

1. In a large pot, heat the olive oil over medium heat. Add the onion and garlic, and cook for 3-4 minutes until softened.
2. Add the broccoli florets, vegetable broth, almond flour, and dried thyme. Bring to a boil.
3. Reduce heat and simmer for 15-20 minutes, or until the broccoli is tender.
4. Stir in the almond milk and cook for another 5 minutes.
5. Use an immersion blender to puree the soup until smooth.
6. Garnish with fresh chives before serving.

Nutrition Info per Serving (Serves 6):

- Calories: 180
- Protein: 5g
- Carbohydrates: 12g
- Fiber: 5g
- Sugars: 3g
- Fat: 13g
- Saturated Fat: 1g

Cooking Time:

- **Total: 30 minutes**

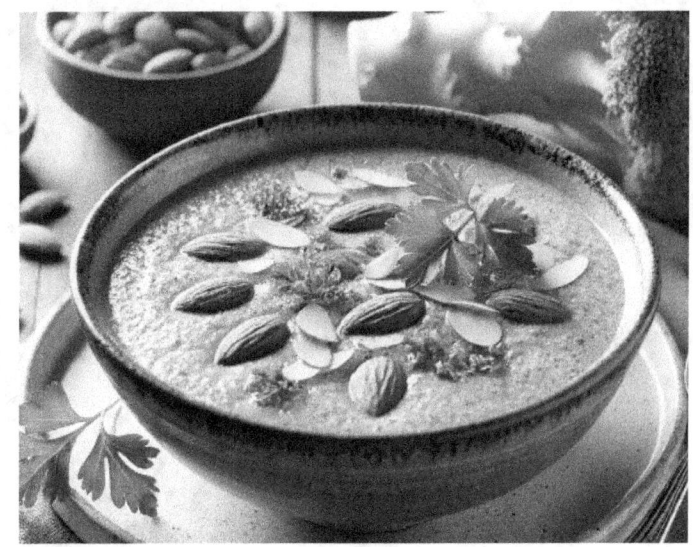

8. Cabbage Soup
Ingredients:
- 2 tablespoons olive oil
- 1 onion, chopped
- 3 cloves garlic, minced
- 4 cups chopped cabbage
- 2 carrots, peeled and sliced
- 2 celery stalks, sliced
- 6 cups low-sodium vegetable broth
- 1 teaspoon dried thyme
- 1 teaspoon dried oregano
- Fresh parsley for garnish

Instructions:
1. In a large pot, heat the olive oil over medium heat. Add the onion and garlic, and cook for 3-4 minutes until softened.
2. Stir in the cabbage, carrots, and celery. Cook for another 5 minutes.
3. Add the vegetable broth, thyme, and oregano. Bring to a boil.
4. Reduce heat and simmer for 25-30 minutes, or until the vegetables are tender.
5. Garnish with fresh parsley before serving.

Nutrition Info per Serving (Serves 6):
- Calories: 120
- Protein: 4g
- Carbohydrates: 18g
- Fiber: 5g
- Sugars: 7g
- Fat: 5g
- Saturated Fat: 1g

Cooking Time:
- **Total: 35 minutes**

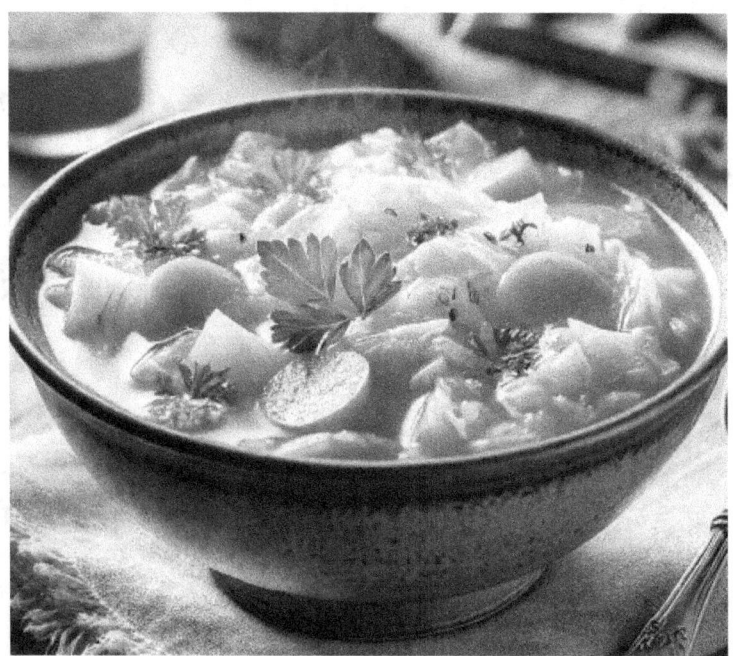

9. Pea Soup with Mint

Ingredients:

- 2 tablespoons olive oil
- 1 onion, chopped
- 3 cloves garlic, minced
- 4 cups frozen peas
- 4 cups low-sodium vegetable broth
- 1/4 cup fresh mint leaves, chopped
- 1/2 cup coconut milk
- Fresh mint leaves for garnish

Instructions:

1. In a large pot, heat the olive oil over medium heat. Add the onion and garlic, and cook for 3-4 minutes until softened.
2. Add the frozen peas and vegetable broth. Bring to a boil.
3. Reduce heat and simmer for 10-15 minutes, or until the peas are tender.
4. Stir in the chopped mint leaves and coconut milk. Cook for another 5 minutes.
5. Use an immersion blender to puree the soup until smooth.
6. Garnish with fresh mint leaves before serving.

Nutrition Info per Serving (Serves 6):

- Calories: 180
- Protein: 5g
- Carbohydrates: 22g
- Fiber: 6g
- Sugars: 7g
- Fat: 9g
- Saturated Fat: 7g

Cooking Time:

- **Total: 25 minutes**

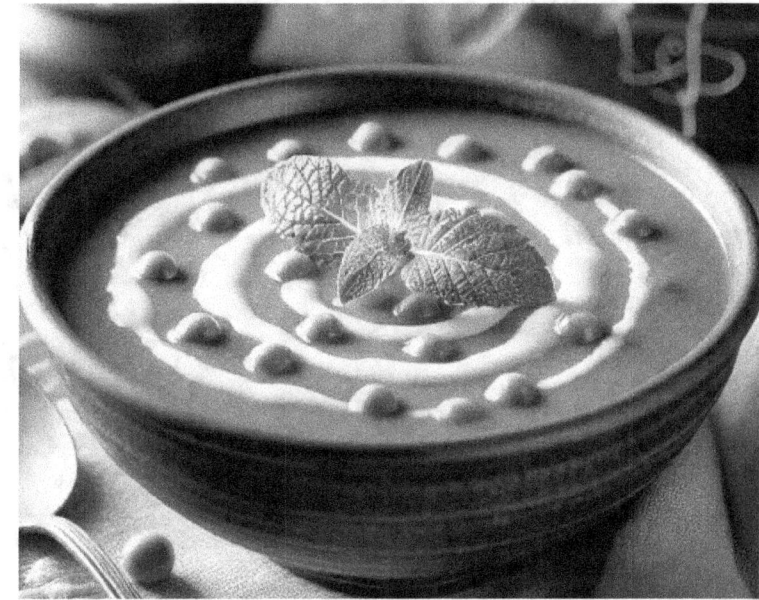

10. Squash and Lentil Stew

Ingredients:

- 2 tablespoons olive oil
- 1 onion, chopped
- 3 cloves garlic, minced
- 2 cups butternut squash, peeled and cubed
- 1 cup dried lentils, rinsed
- 6 cups low-sodium vegetable broth
- 1 teaspoon ground cumin
- 1 teaspoon ground coriander
- 1 teaspoon ground turmeric
- 1 cup chopped tomatoes (fresh or canned)
- Fresh cilantro for garnish

Instructions:

1. In a large pot, heat the olive oil over medium heat. Add the onion and garlic, and cook for 3-4 minutes until softened.
2. Add the butternut squash, lentils, vegetable broth, cumin, coriander, and turmeric. Bring to a boil.
3. Reduce heat and simmer for 25-30 minutes, or until the lentils and squash are tender.
4. Stir in the chopped tomatoes and cook for another 5 minutes.
5. Garnish with fresh cilantro before serving.

Nutrition Info per Serving (Serves 6):

- Calories: 250
- Protein: 10g
- Carbohydrates: 40g
- Fiber: 12g
- Sugars: 8g
- Fat: 7g
- Saturated Fat: 1g

Cooking Time:

- **Total: 40 minutes**

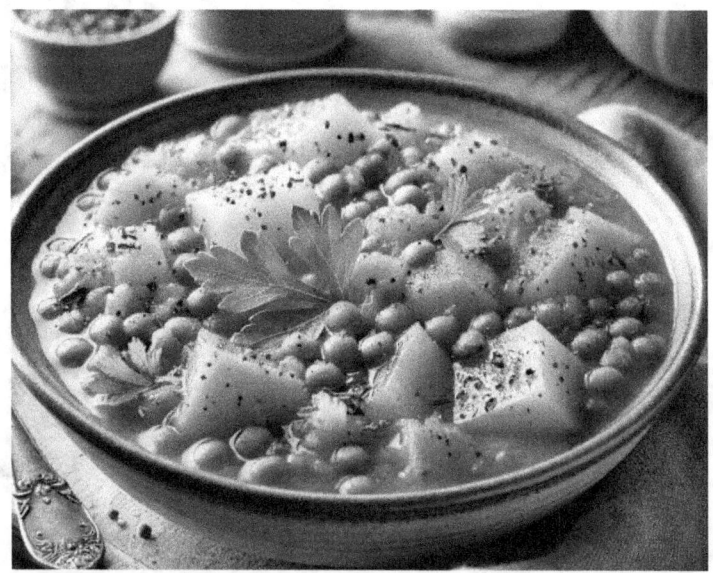

11. Turkey and Sweet Potato Soup

Ingredients:

- 2 tablespoons olive oil
- 1 onion, chopped
- 3 cloves garlic, minced
- 1 pound ground turkey
- 2 large sweet potatoes, peeled and cubed
- 6 cups low-sodium chicken broth
- 1 teaspoon dried thyme
- 1 teaspoon dried rosemary
- 2 cups chopped kale
- 1 lemon, juiced

Instructions:

1. In a large pot, heat the olive oil over medium heat. Add the onion and garlic, and cook for 3-4 minutes until softened.
2. Add the ground turkey and cook until browned, about 5-7 minutes.
3. Stir in the sweet potatoes, chicken broth, thyme, and rosemary. Bring to a boil.
4. Reduce heat and simmer for 20-25 minutes, or until the sweet potatoes are tender.
5. Stir in the chopped kale and cook for another 5 minutes until wilted.
6. Add lemon juice before serving.

Nutrition Info per Serving (Serves 6):

- Calories: 280
- Protein: 25g
- Carbohydrates: 30g
- Fiber: 6g
- Sugars: 8g
- Fat: 10g
- Saturated Fat: 2g

Cooking Time:

- **Total: 40 minutes**

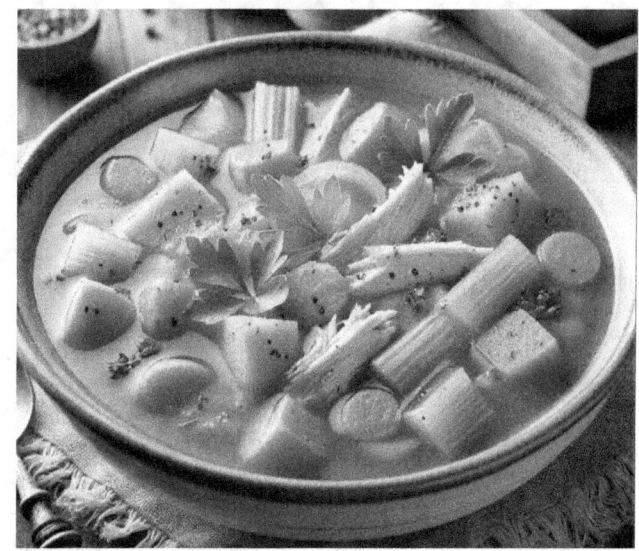

12. Beet Soup with Dill

Ingredients:

- 2 tablespoons olive oil
- 1 onion, chopped
- 3 cloves garlic, minced
- 4 large beets, peeled and diced
- 4 cups low-sodium vegetable broth
- 1 teaspoon dried dill
- 1 cup coconut milk
- 1 lemon, juiced
- Fresh dill for garnish

Instructions:

1. In a large pot, heat the olive oil over medium heat. Add the onion and garlic, and cook for 3-4 minutes until softened.
2. Add the diced beets and vegetable broth. Bring to a boil.
3. Reduce heat and simmer for 30-35 minutes, or until the beets are tender.
4. Stir in the dried dill and coconut milk. Cook for another 5 minutes.
5. Use an immersion blender to puree the soup until smooth.
6. Add lemon juice before serving and garnish with fresh dill.

Nutrition Info per Serving (Serves 6):

- Calories: 220
- Protein: 3g
- Carbohydrates: 25g
- Fiber: 6g
- Sugars: 15g
- Fat: 12g
- Saturated Fat: 8g

Cooking Time:

- **Total: 45 minutes**

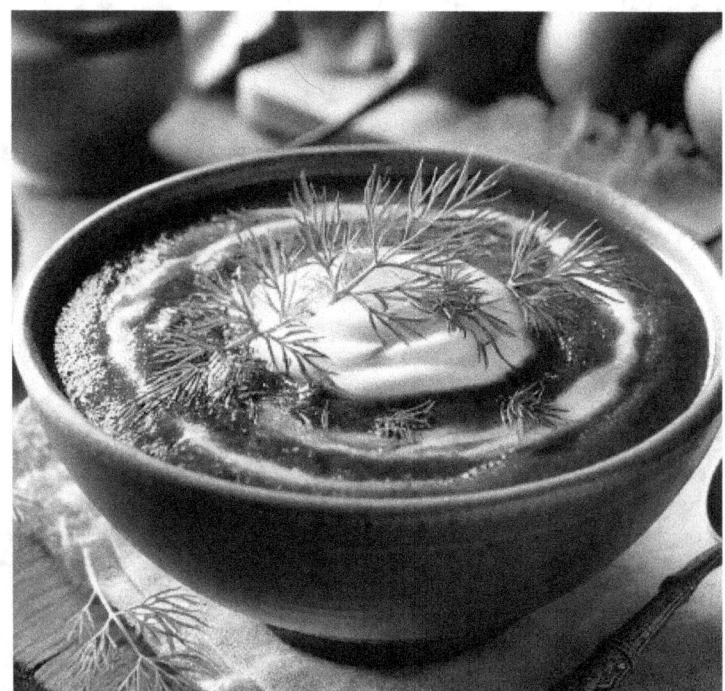

13. Leek and Potato Soup

Ingredients:

- 2 tablespoons olive oil
- 3 leeks, white and light green parts only, sliced
- 3 cloves garlic, minced
- 4 large potatoes, peeled and diced
- 6 cups low-sodium vegetable broth
- 1 teaspoon dried thyme
- 1 cup coconut milk
- Fresh chives for garnish

Instructions:

1. In a large pot, heat the olive oil over medium heat. Add the leeks and garlic, and cook for 5-7 minutes until softened.
2. Stir in the diced potatoes, vegetable broth, and thyme. Bring to a boil.
3. Reduce heat and simmer for 20-25 minutes, or until the potatoes are tender.
4. Stir in the coconut milk and cook for another 5 minutes.
5. Use an immersion blender to puree the soup until smooth.
6. Garnish with fresh chives before serving.

Nutrition Info per Serving (Serves 6):

- Calories: 250
- Protein: 4g
- Carbohydrates: 40g
- Fiber: 5g
- Sugars: 4g
- Fat: 10g
- Saturated Fat: 7g

Cooking Time:

- **Total: 35 minutes**

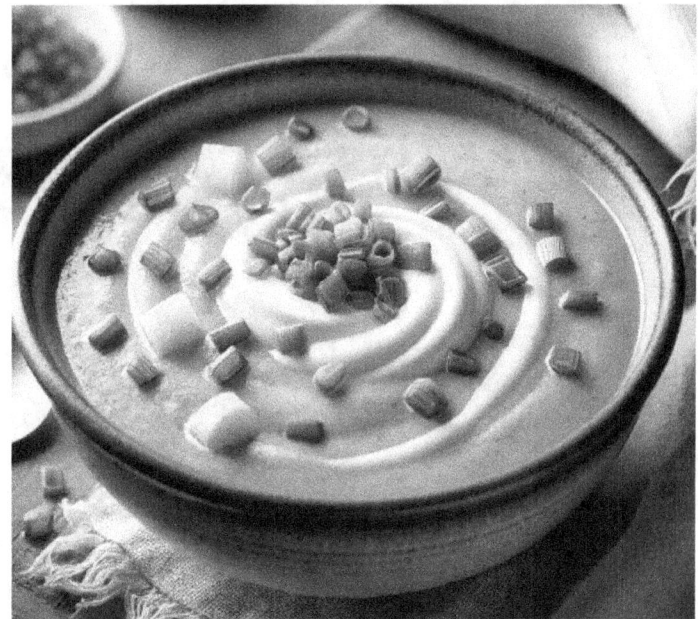

14. Quinoa Vegetable Soup

Ingredients:

- 2 tablespoons olive oil
- 1 onion, chopped
- 3 cloves garlic, minced
- 2 carrots, peeled and sliced
- 2 celery stalks, sliced
- 1 cup quinoa, rinsed
- 6 cups low-sodium vegetable broth
- 1 teaspoon dried oregano
- 1 teaspoon dried basil
- 2 cups chopped kale
- 1 lemon, juiced

Instructions:

1. In a large pot, heat the olive oil over medium heat. Add the onion and garlic, and cook for 3-4 minutes until softened.
2. Stir in the carrots, celery, and quinoa. Cook for another 5 minutes.
3. Add the vegetable broth, oregano, and basil. Bring to a boil.
4. Reduce heat and simmer for 15-20 minutes, or until the quinoa is cooked and the vegetables are tender.
5. Stir in the chopped kale and cook for another 5 minutes until wilted.
6. Add lemon juice before serving.

Nutrition Info per Serving (Serves 6):

- Calories: 220
- Protein: 7g
- Carbohydrates: 35g
- Fiber: 7g
- Sugars: 6g
- Fat: 7g
- Saturated Fat: 1g

Cooking Time:

- **Total: 35 minutes**

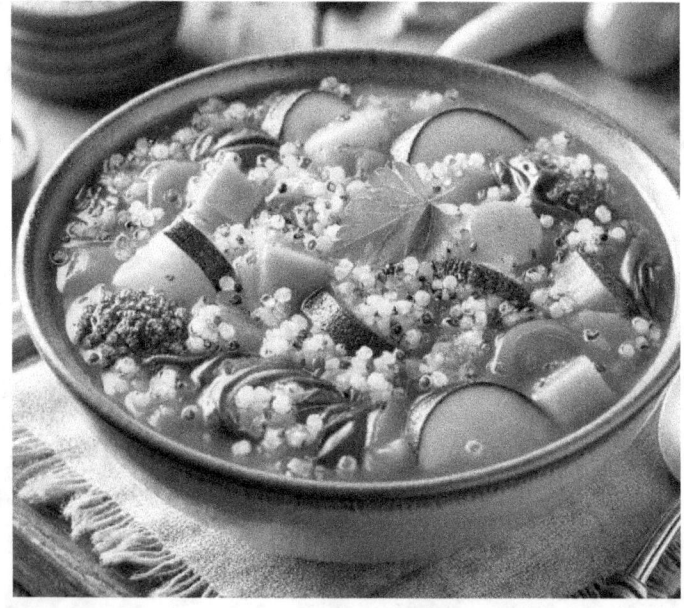

15. Chickpea and Spinach Stew

Ingredients:

- 2 tablespoons olive oil
- 1 onion, chopped
- 3 cloves garlic, minced
- 2 cans (15 oz each) chickpeas, drained and rinsed
- 1 can (14.5 oz) diced tomatoes, no salt added
- 4 cups low-sodium vegetable broth
- 1 teaspoon ground cumin
- 1 teaspoon ground coriander
- 1 teaspoon smoked paprika
- 4 cups fresh spinach
- Fresh cilantro for garnish

Instructions:

1. In a large pot, heat the olive oil over medium heat. Add the onion and garlic, and cook for 3-4 minutes until softened.
2. Stir in the chickpeas, diced tomatoes, vegetable broth, cumin, coriander, and smoked paprika. Bring to a boil.
3. Reduce heat and simmer for 20-25 minutes, allowing the flavors to meld.
4. Stir in the fresh spinach and cook for another 5 minutes until wilted.
5. Garnish with fresh cilantro before serving.

Nutrition Info per Serving (Serves 6):

- Calories: 240
- Protein: 10g
- Carbohydrates: 35g
- Fiber: 10g
- Sugars: 8g
- Fat: 7g
- Saturated Fat: 1g

Cooking Time:

- **Total: 35 minutes**

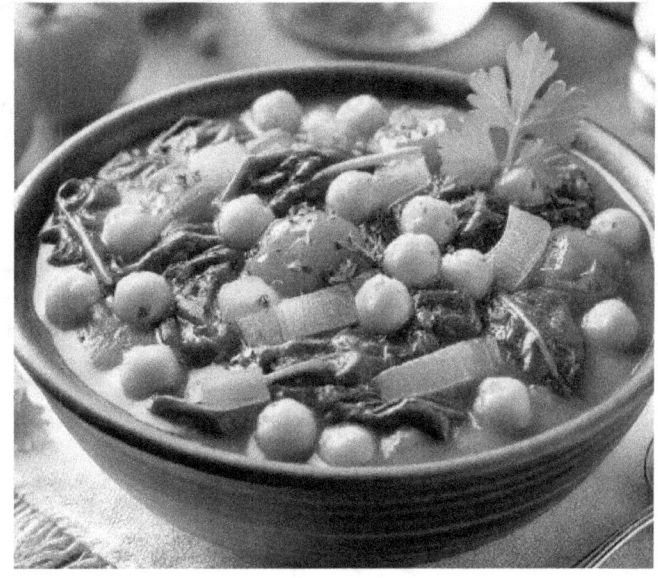

16. Celery Soup with Garlic

Ingredients:

- 2 tablespoons olive oil
- 1 onion, chopped
- 3 cloves garlic, minced
- 6 cups chopped celery (about 1 bunch)
- 4 cups low-sodium vegetable broth
- 1 teaspoon dried thyme
- 1 cup coconut milk
- Fresh parsley for garnish

Instructions:

1. In a large pot, heat the olive oil over medium heat. Add the onion and garlic, and cook for 3-4 minutes until softened.
2. Add the chopped celery, vegetable broth, and thyme. Bring to a boil.
3. Reduce heat and simmer for 20-25 minutes, or until the celery is tender.
4. Stir in the coconut milk and cook for another 5 minutes.
5. Use an immersion blender to puree the soup until smooth.
6. Garnish with fresh parsley before serving.

Nutrition Info per Serving (Serves 6):

- Calories: 180
- Protein: 3g
- Carbohydrates: 15g
- Fiber: 4g
- Sugars: 5g
- Fat: 12g
- Saturated Fat: 7g

Cooking Time:

- **Total: 30 minutes**

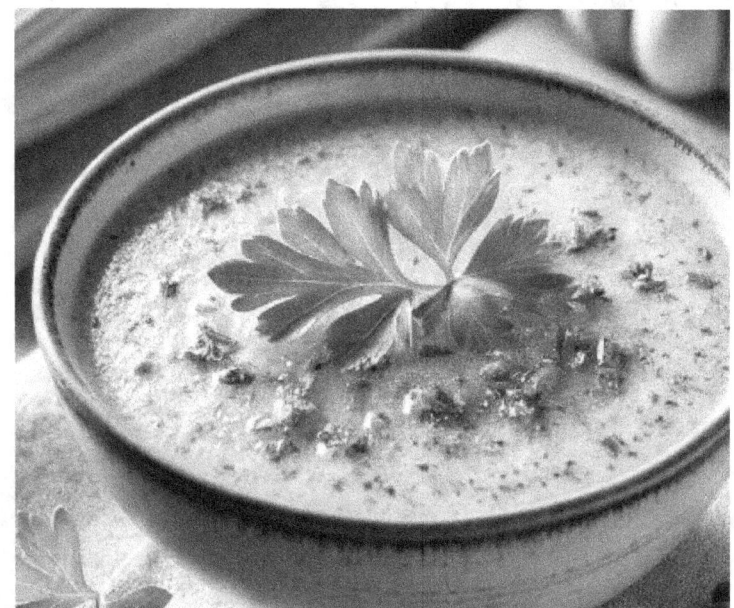

17. Kimchi Stew with Tofu
Ingredients:

- 2 tablespoons olive oil
- 1 onion, chopped
- 3 cloves garlic, minced
- 2 cups kimchi, chopped
- 4 cups low-sodium vegetable broth
- 1 tablespoon gochujang (Korean red chili paste)
- 1 block (14 oz) firm tofu, cubed
- 1 teaspoon sesame oil
- 2 green onions, sliced

Instructions:

1. In a large pot, heat the olive oil over medium heat. Add the onion and garlic, and cook for 3-4 minutes until softened.
2. Stir in the kimchi and gochujang. Cook for another 3-4 minutes.
3. Add the vegetable broth and bring to a boil.
4. Reduce heat and simmer for 15 minutes.
5. Add the cubed tofu and cook for another 5 minutes until heated through.
6. Stir in the sesame oil.
7. Garnish with sliced green onions before serving.

Nutrition Info per Serving (Serves 4):

- Calories: 200
- Protein: 10g
- Carbohydrates: 12g
- Fiber: 3g
- Sugars: 4g
- Fat: 14g
- Saturated Fat: 2g

Cooking Time:

- **Total: 30 minutes**

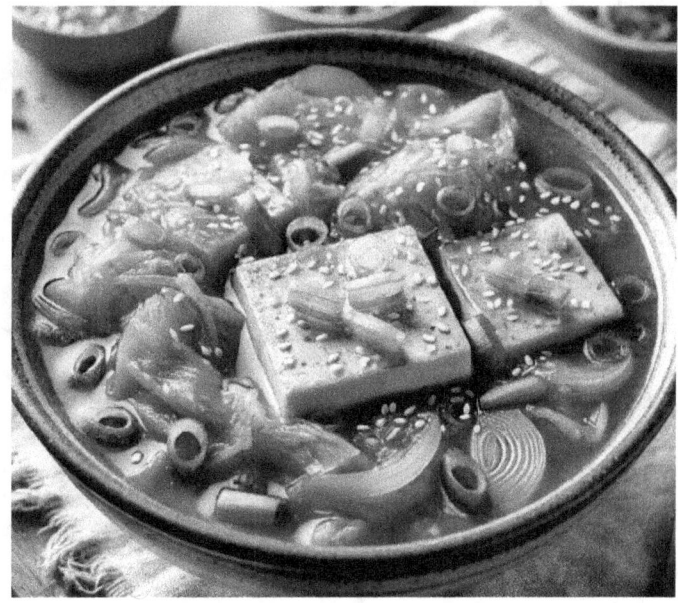

18. Saffron and Seafood Stew

Ingredients:

- 2 tablespoons olive oil
- 1 onion, chopped
- 3 cloves garlic, minced
- 1 red bell pepper, chopped
- 1 can (14.5 oz) diced tomatoes, no salt added
- 4 cups low-sodium fish broth
- 1/4 teaspoon saffron threads
- 1 pound white fish fillets, cut into chunks
- 1/2 pound shrimp, peeled and deveined
- 1/2 pound mussels, scrubbed and debearded
- 1/4 cup fresh parsley, chopped

Instructions:

1. In a large pot, heat the olive oil over medium heat. Add the onion, garlic, and red bell pepper, and cook for 5-7 minutes until softened.
2. Stir in the diced tomatoes, fish broth, and saffron threads. Bring to a boil.
3. Reduce heat and simmer for 10 minutes.
4. Add the white fish fillets, shrimp, and mussels. Cook for another 5-7 minutes until the seafood is cooked through and the mussels open. Discard any mussels that do not open.
5. Garnish with fresh parsley before serving.

Nutrition Info per Serving (Serves 4):

- Calories: 300
- Protein: 30g
- Carbohydrates: 10g
- Fiber: 2g
- Sugars: 4g
- Fat: 12g
- Saturated Fat: 2g

Cooking Time:

- **Total: 30 minutes**

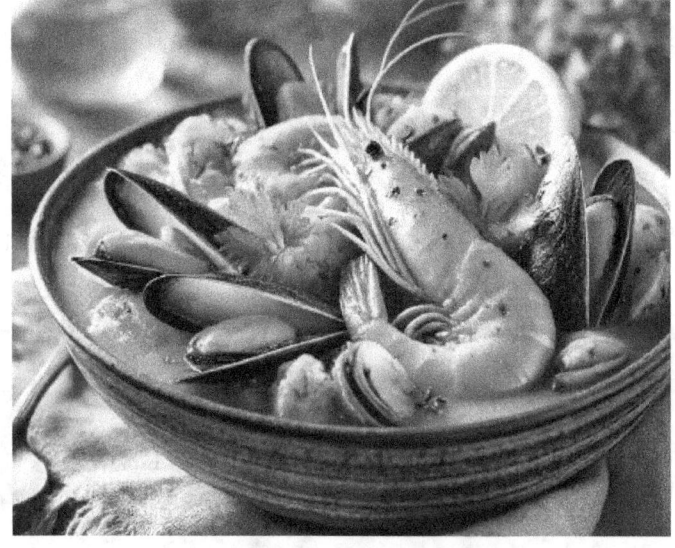

19. Bean and Escarole Soup

Ingredients:

- 2 tablespoons olive oil
- 1 onion, chopped
- 3 cloves garlic, minced
- 2 carrots, peeled and sliced
- 2 cans (15 oz each) cannellini beans, drained and rinsed
- 6 cups low-sodium vegetable broth
- 1 teaspoon dried thyme
- 1 head escarole, chopped
- 1 lemon, juiced

Instructions:

1. In a large pot, heat the olive oil over medium heat. Add the onion, garlic, and carrots, and cook for 5-7 minutes until softened.
2. Stir in the cannellini beans, vegetable broth, and thyme. Bring to a boil.
3. Reduce heat and simmer for 20 minutes.
4. Add the chopped escarole and cook for another 5 minutes until wilted.
5. Add lemon juice before serving.

Nutrition Info per Serving (Serves 6):

- Calories: 220
- Protein: 10g
- Carbohydrates: 35g
- Fiber: 10g
- Sugars: 6g
- Fat: 6g
- Saturated Fat: 1g

Cooking Time:

- **Total: 35 minutes**

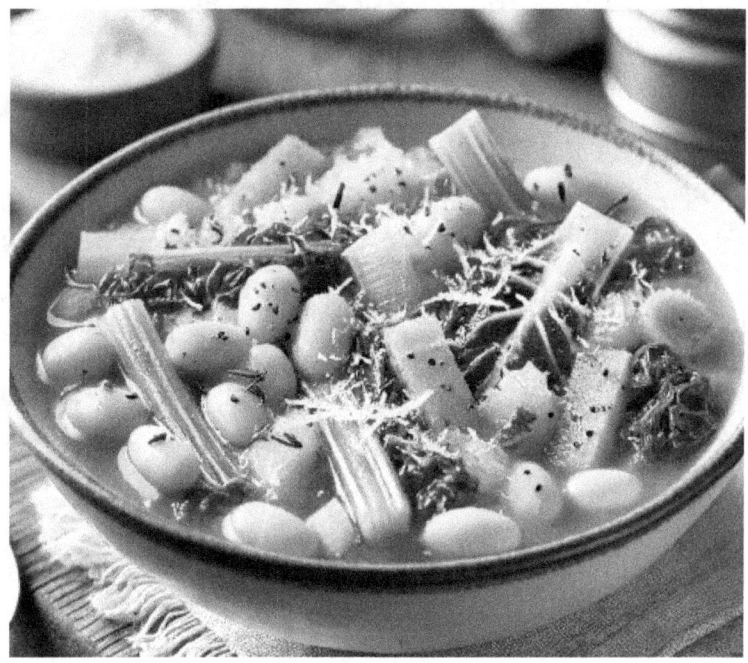

20. Bok Choy and Shiitake Mushroom Soup

Ingredients:

- 2 tablespoons olive oil
- 1 onion, chopped
- 3 cloves garlic, minced
- 1 tablespoon fresh ginger, grated
- 6 cups low-sodium vegetable broth
- 1 cup sliced shiitake mushrooms
- 4 cups chopped bok choy
- 2 tablespoons low-sodium soy sauce
- 2 green onions, sliced

Instructions:

1. In a large pot, heat the olive oil over medium heat. Add the onion, garlic, and ginger, and cook for 3-4 minutes until softened.
2. Stir in the vegetable broth and bring to a boil.
3. Add the shiitake mushrooms and cook for 5-7 minutes until tender.
4. Stir in the chopped bok choy and soy sauce. Cook for another 5 minutes until the bok choy is wilted.
5. Garnish with sliced green onions before serving.

Nutrition Info per Serving (Serves 4):

- Calories: 150
- Protein: 5g
- Carbohydrates: 18g
- Fiber: 5g
- Sugars: 6g
- Fat: 7g
- Saturated Fat: 1g

Cooking Time:

- **Total: 25 minutes**

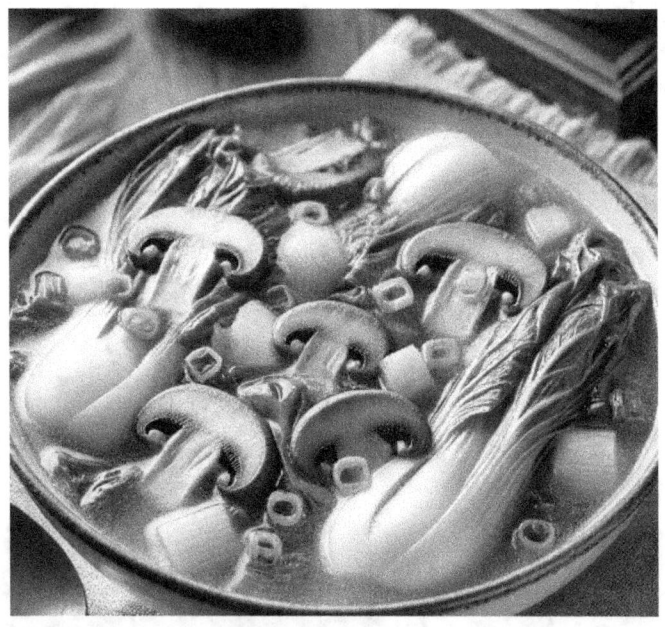

10-WEEK MEAL PLAN

Week 1
Monday
- Breakfast: Oatmeal with Chopped Apples and Cinnamon
- Lunch: Grilled Chicken with Herb Salad
- Dinner: Beef Stir Fry with Broccoli

Tuesday
- Breakfast: Smoothie Bowl with Berries and Seeds
- Lunch: Chicken and Broccoli Stir-Fry
- Dinner: Lamb and Spinach Curry

Wednesday
- Breakfast: Buckwheat Pancakes
- Lunch: Turkey and Sweet Potato Skillet
- Dinner: Baked Cod with Parsley Pesto

Thursday
- Breakfast: Sweet Potato Hash
- Lunch: Seared Scallops with Cauliflower Puree
- Dinner: Pumpkin Soup with Nutmeg

Friday
- Breakfast: Quinoa Porridge
- Lunch: Grilled Tuna Steaks with Avocado Salsa
- Dinner: Saffron and Seafood Stew

Saturday
- Breakfast: Banana Almond Smoothie
- Lunch: Chicken Apple Sausages
- Dinner: Lentil Soup with Kale

Sunday
- Breakfast: Rice Cakes with Almond Butter and Banana Slices
- Lunch: Poached Halibut with Dill Sauce
- Dinner: Spiced Lamb Kebabs

Week 2
Monday
- Breakfast: Baked Oatmeal Cups
- Lunch: Turkey Meatloaf
- Dinner: Clam Soup with Vegetables

Tuesday
- Breakfast: Kale and Apple Smoothie
- Lunch: Rosemary Chicken Skewers
- Dinner: Spinach and White Bean Soup

Wednesday
- Breakfast: Homemade Granola
- Lunch: Grilled Sirloin Steak with Asparagus
- Dinner: Carrot and Coriander Soup

Thursday
- Breakfast: Pumpkin Spice Porridge
- Lunch: One-Pan Turmeric Chicken and Rice
- Dinner: Sea Bass with Fennel and Orange

Friday
- Breakfast: Sautéed Vegetables and Quinoa
- Lunch: Slow Cooker Turkey Soup
- Dinner: Lamb Chops with Cauliflower Rice

Saturday
- Breakfast: Berry and Walnut Salad
- Lunch: Beef and Squash Stew
- Dinner: Pea Soup with Mint

Sunday
- Breakfast: Almond Flour Muffins
- Lunch: Balsamic Glazed Turkey Breast
- Dinner: Quinoa Vegetable Soup

Week 3

Monday
- Breakfast: Spinach and Mushroom Omelette
- Lunch: Chicken Vegetable Kabobs
- Dinner: Beet Soup with Dill

Tuesday
- Breakfast: Savory Buckwheat Crepes
- Lunch: Turkey Spinach Mini Meatballs
- Dinner: Squash and Lentil Stew

Wednesday
- Breakfast: Pineapple and Spinach Green Juice
- Lunch: Grilled Lamb Chops with Mint Pesto
- Dinner: Celery Soup with Garlic

Thursday
- Breakfast: Herbed Chicken Patties
- Lunch: Beef Kabobs with Bell Peppers
- Dinner: Kimchi Stew with Tofu

Friday
- Breakfast: Green Tea with Lemon and Honey
- Lunch: Turkey and Kale Soup
- Dinner: Bean and Escarole Soup

Saturday
- Breakfast: Flaxseed and Banana Pancakes
- Lunch: Pork Stir Fry with Snow Peas
- Dinner: Bok Choy and Shiitake Mushroom Soup

Sunday
- Breakfast: Kefir with Honey and Almonds
- Lunch: Lamb Stir Fry with Zucchini
- Dinner: Beef Tomato Stew

Week 4

Monday
- Breakfast: Oatmeal with Chopped Apples and Cinnamon
- Lunch: Turkey Meatloaf
- Dinner: Beef Bone Broth

Tuesday
- Breakfast: Smoothie Bowl with Berries and Seeds
- Lunch: Chicken Soup with Vegetables
- Dinner: Lamb Tagine with Apricots

Wednesday
- Breakfast: Buckwheat Pancakes
- Lunch: Grilled Sirloin Steak with Asparagus
- Dinner: Broccoli and Almond Soup

Thursday
- Breakfast: Sweet Potato Hash
- Lunch: Grilled Tuna Steaks with Avocado Salsa
- Dinner: Cabbage Soup

Friday
- Breakfast: Quinoa Porridge
- Lunch: Seared Tuna with Sesame Seeds
- Dinner: Clam and Spinach Pasta

Saturday
- Breakfast: Banana Almond Smoothie
- Lunch: One-Pan Turmeric Chicken and Rice
- Dinner: Chickpea and Spinach Stew

Sunday
- Breakfast: Rice Cakes with Almond Butter and Banana Slices
- Lunch: Baked Cod with Parsley Pesto
- Dinner: Flounder with Herb Crust

Week 5

Monday
- Breakfast: Baked Oatmeal Cups
- Lunch: Chicken Apple Sausages
- Dinner: Grilled Branzino with Lemon Butter

Tuesday
- Breakfast: Kale and Apple Smoothie
- Lunch: Rosemary Chicken Skewers
- Dinner: Lentil Soup with Kale

Wednesday
- Breakfast: Homemade Granola
- Lunch: Balsamic Glazed Turkey Breast
- Dinner: Leek and Potato Soup

Thursday
- Breakfast: Pumpkin Spice Porridge
- Lunch: Turkey and Sweet Potato Skillet
- Dinner: Anchovy and Green Bean Salad

Friday
- Breakfast: Sautéed Vegetables and Quinoa
- Lunch: Grilled Lamb Chops with Mint Pesto
- Dinner: Saffron and Seafood Stew

Saturday
- Breakfast: Berry and Walnut Salad
- Lunch: Grilled Chicken with Herb Salad
- Dinner: Monkfish with Tomato and Capers

Sunday
- Breakfast: Almond Flour Muffins
- Lunch: Seared Scallops with Cauliflower Puree
- Dinner: Bean and Escarole Soup

Week 6

Monday
- Breakfast: Kale and Apple Smoothie
- Lunch: Lamb Salad with Mixed Greens
- Dinner: Miso Soup with Tofu and Seaweed

Tuesday
- Breakfast: Homemade Granola
- Lunch: Herb-Roasted Chicken Breast
- Dinner: Broccoli and Almond Soup

Wednesday
- Breakfast: Pumpkin Spice Porridge
- Lunch: Grilled Beef Salad with Arugula
- Dinner: Beet Soup with Dill

Thursday
- Breakfast: Pineapple and Spinach Green Juice
- Lunch: Baked Trout with Almonds
- Dinner: Carrot and Coriander Soup

Friday
- Breakfast: Herbed Chicken Patties
- Lunch: Beef and Green Bean Salad
- Dinner: Cabbage Soup

Saturday
- Breakfast: Green Tea with Lemon and Honey
- Lunch: Turkey and Spinach Stuffed Mushrooms
- Dinner: Leek and Potato Soup

Sunday
- Breakfast: Flaxseed and Banana Pancakes
- Lunch: Poached Chicken with Avocado Salsa
- Dinner: Saffron and Seafood Stew

Week 7

Monday
- Breakfast: Kefir with Honey and Almonds
- Lunch: Turkey and Sweet Potato Skillet
- Dinner: Lentil Soup with Kale

Tuesday
- Breakfast: Oatmeal with Chopped Apples and Cinnamon
- Lunch: Lamb Chops with Cauliflower Rice
- Dinner: Squash and Lentil Stew

Wednesday
- Breakfast: Smoothie Bowl with Berries and Seeds
- Lunch: Chicken Vegetable Kabobs
- Dinner: Celery Soup with Garlic

Thursday
- Breakfast: Buckwheat Pancakes
- Lunch: Balsamic Glazed Turkey Breast
- Dinner: Kimchi Stew with Tofu

Friday
- Breakfast: Sweet Potato Hash
- Lunch: Grilled Swordfish with Basil Oil
- Dinner: Bean and Escarole Soup

Saturday
- Breakfast: Quinoa Porridge
- Lunch: Pork Tenderloin with Cherry Sauce
- Dinner: Bok Choy and Shiitake Mushroom Soup

Sunday
- Breakfast: Banana Almond Smoothie
- Lunch: Tilapia with Mango Salsa
- Dinner: Clam and Spinach Pasta

Week 8

Monday
- Breakfast: Rice Cakes with Almond Butter and Banana Slices
- Lunch: Lamb Stir Fry with Zucchini
- Dinner: Beet Soup with Dill

Tuesday
- Breakfast: Baked Oatmeal Cups
- Lunch: Turkey Spinach Mini Meatballs
- Dinner: Pea Soup with Mint

Wednesday
- Breakfast: Kale and Apple Smoothie
- Lunch: Grilled Salmon with Dill and Lemon
- Dinner: Cabbage Soup

Thursday
- Breakfast: Homemade Granola
- Lunch: Poached Halibut with Dill Sauce
- Dinner: Leek and Potato Soup

Friday
- Breakfast: Pumpkin Spice Porridge
- Lunch: One-Pan Turmeric Chicken and Rice
- Dinner: Chickpea and Spinach Stew

Saturday
- Breakfast: Sautéed Vegetables and Quinoa
- Lunch: Grilled Lamb Chops with Mint Pesto
- Dinner: Carrot and Coriander Soup

Sunday
- Breakfast: Berry and Walnut Salad
- Lunch: Turkey and Sweet Potato Soup
- Dinner: Kimchi Stew with Tofu

Week 9

Monday
- Breakfast: Almond Flour Muffins
- Lunch: Beef Stir Fry with Broccoli
- Dinner: Squash and Lentil Stew

Tuesday
- Breakfast: Spinach and Mushroom Omelette
- Lunch: Grilled Branzino with Lemon Butter
- Dinner: Lentil Soup with Kale

Wednesday
- Breakfast: Savory Buckwheat Crepes
- Lunch: Turkey and Spinach Stuffed Mushrooms
- Dinner: Celery Soup with Garlic

Thursday
- Breakfast: Pineapple and Spinach Green Juice
- Lunch: Pork Stir Fry with Snow Peas
- Dinner: Cabbage Soup

Friday
- Breakfast: Herbed Chicken Patties
- Lunch: Beef Kabobs with Bell Peppers
- Dinner: Beet Soup with Dill

Saturday
- Breakfast: Green Tea with Lemon and Honey
- Lunch: Seared Tuna with Sesame Seeds
- Dinner: Bok Choy and Shiitake Mushroom Soup

Sunday
- Breakfast: Flaxseed and Banana Pancakes
- Lunch: Chicken Soup with Vegetables
- Dinner: Bean and Escarole Soup

Week 10

Monday
- Breakfast: Kefir with Honey and Almonds
- Lunch: Grilled Chicken with Herb Salad
- Dinner: Pea Soup with Mint

Tuesday
- Breakfast: Oatmeal with Chopped Apples and Cinnamon
- Lunch: Grilled Sirloin Steak with Asparagus
- Dinner: Kimchi Stew with Tofu

Wednesday
- Breakfast: Smoothie Bowl with Berries and Seeds
- Lunch: Baked Trout with Almonds
- Dinner: Celery Soup with Garlic

Thursday
- Breakfast: Buckwheat Pancakes
- Lunch: Tilapia with Mango Salsa
- Dinner: Leek and Potato Soup

Friday
- Breakfast: Sweet Potato Hash
- Lunch: Lamb Salad with Mixed Greens
- Dinner: Squash and Lentil Stew

Saturday
- Breakfast: Quinoa Porridge
- Lunch: Grilled Swordfish with Basil Oil
- Dinner: Saffron and Seafood Stew

Sunday
- Breakfast: Banana Almond Smoothie
- Lunch: Beef and Green Bean Salad
- Dinner: Lentil Soup with Kale

WEEKLY MEAL PLANNER + WORKBOOK

	BREAKFAST	LUNCH	DINNER	SNACKS
MONDAY				
TUESDAY				
WEDNESDAY				
THURSDAY				
FRIDAY				
SATURDAY				
SUNDAY				

What are your personal goals for starting the CRPS diet? How do you hope it will help manage your symptoms?

....

....

....

....

....

....

WEEKLY MEAL PLANNER + WORKBOOK

	BREAKFAST	LUNCH	DINNER	SNACKS
MONDAY				
TUESDAY				
WEDNESDAY				
THURSDAY				
FRIDAY				
SATURDAY				
SUNDAY				

Describe your current diet. What foods do you eat regularly, and how do you feel after eating them?

....

....

....

....

....

....

WEEKLY MEAL PLANNER + WORKBOOK

	BREAKFAST	LUNCH	DINNER	SNACKS
MONDAY				
TUESDAY				
WEDNESDAY				
THURSDAY				
FRIDAY				
SATURDAY				
SUNDAY				

What are the biggest changes you will need to make to follow the CRPS diet? How do you feel about these changes?

....

....

....

....

....

....

WEEKLY MEAL PLANNER + WORKBOOK

	BREAKFAST	LUNCH	DINNER	SNACKS
MONDAY				
TUESDAY				
WEDNESDAY				
THURSDAY				
FRIDAY				
SATURDAY				
SUNDAY				

How do you plan to incorporate more anti-inflammatory foods into your meals? List three specific changes you can make.

....

....

....

....

....

....

WEEKLY MEAL PLANNER + WORKBOOK

	BREAKFAST	LUNCH	DINNER	SNACKS
MONDAY				
TUESDAY				
WEDNESDAY				
THURSDAY				
FRIDAY				
SATURDAY				
SUNDAY				

Which CRPS-friendly foods are you most excited to try? Why?

....

....

....

....

....

....

WEEKLY MEAL PLANNER + WORKBOOK

	BREAKFAST	LUNCH	DINNER	SNACKS
MONDAY				
TUESDAY				
WEDNESDAY				
THURSDAY				
FRIDAY				
SATURDAY				
SUNDAY				

What challenges do you anticipate in following the CRPS diet? What strategies can you use to overcome these challenges?

....

....

....

....

....

....

WEEKLY MEAL PLANNER + WORKBOOK

	BREAKFAST	LUNCH	DINNER	SNACKS
MONDAY				
TUESDAY				
WEDNESDAY				
THURSDAY				
FRIDAY				
SATURDAY				
SUNDAY				

Who can support you in making dietary changes? How can they help you stay on track?

....

....

....

....

....

....

WEEKLY MEAL PLANNER + WORKBOOK

	BREAKFAST	LUNCH	DINNER	SNACKS
MONDAY				
TUESDAY				
WEDNESDAY				
THURSDAY				
FRIDAY				
SATURDAY				
SUNDAY				

Create a shopping list of CRPS-friendly foods you need to buy for the week. How will you ensure you stick to this list?

....

....

....

....

....

....

WEEKLY MEAL PLANNER + WORKBOOK

	BREAKFAST	LUNCH	DINNER	SNACKS
MONDAY				
TUESDAY				
WEDNESDAY				
THURSDAY				
FRIDAY				
SATURDAY				
SUNDAY				

What new cooking skills do you need to develop to prepare CRPS-friendly meals? How will you learn these skills?

....

....

....

....

....

....

WEEKLY MEAL PLANNER + WORKBOOK

	BREAKFAST	LUNCH	DINNER	SNACKS
MONDAY				
TUESDAY				
WEDNESDAY				
THURSDAY				
FRIDAY				
SATURDAY				
SUNDAY				

How will you handle eating out or social situations where CRPS-friendly options may not be available?

....

....

....

....

....

....

WEEKLY MEAL PLANNER + WORKBOOK

	BREAKFAST	LUNCH	DINNER	SNACKS
MONDAY				
TUESDAY				
WEDNESDAY				
THURSDAY				
FRIDAY				
SATURDAY				
SUNDAY				

How can you practice mindful eating to better understand how different foods affect your body?

....

....

....

....

....

....

WEEKLY MEAL PLANNER + WORKBOOK

	BREAKFAST	LUNCH	DINNER	SNACKS
MONDAY				
TUESDAY				
WEDNESDAY				
THURSDAY				
FRIDAY				
SATURDAY				
SUNDAY				

Which CRPS-friendly recipes have you tried and enjoyed? Why do you like them?

....

....

....

....

....

....

WEEKLY MEAL PLANNER + WORKBOOK

	BREAKFAST	LUNCH	DINNER	SNACKS
MONDAY				
TUESDAY				
WEDNESDAY				
THURSDAY				
FRIDAY				
SATURDAY				
SUNDAY				

How much water do you drink daily? How can staying hydrated support your CRPS diet?

....

....

....

....

....

....

WEEKLY MEAL PLANNER + WORKBOOK

	BREAKFAST	LUNCH	DINNER	SNACKS
MONDAY				
TUESDAY				
WEDNESDAY				
THURSDAY				
FRIDAY				
SATURDAY				
SUNDAY				

How will you track your progress on the CRPS diet? What specific signs will indicate that the diet is helping to manage your symptoms?

....

....

....

....

....

....

Scan the QR code below to get a surprise bonus!

www.ingramcontent.com/pod-product-compliance
Lightning Source LLC
Chambersburg PA
CBHW082234220526
45479CB00005B/1230